AF605582

Sometimes Hearts Have to Break

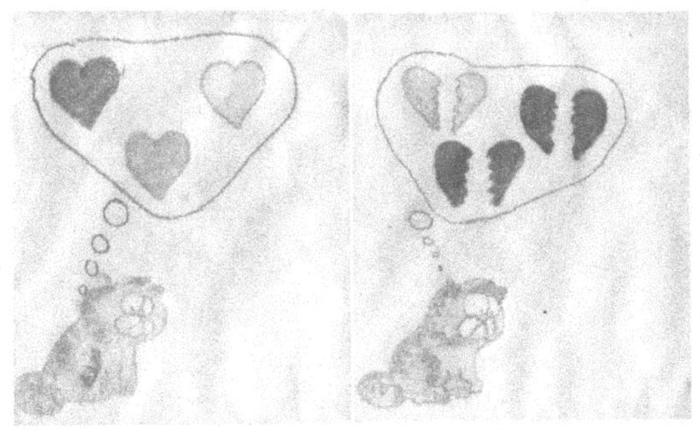

Sometimes Hearts Have to Break

25 Inspirational Journeys to Healing and Peace

Petrea King

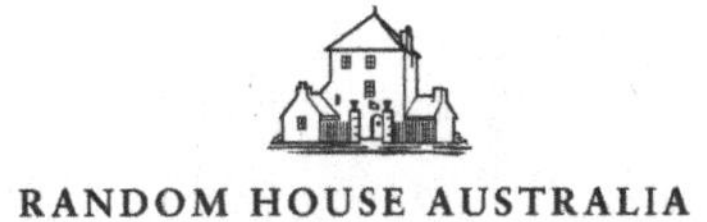

RANDOM HOUSE AUSTRALIA

Random House Australia Pty Ltd
Level 3, 100 Pacific Highway, North Sydney NSW 2060
http://www.randomhouse.com.au

Sydney New York Toronto
London Auckland Johannesburg

First published by Random House Australia in 1997
This edition first published in 2004

Copyright © Petrea King 1997

All rights reserved. No part of this publication may be reproduced, stored in a retrieval system, or transmitted in any form or by any means, electronic, mechanical, photocopying, recording or otherwise, without the prior written permission of the publisher.

National Library of Australia
Cataloguing-in-Publication Entry

King, Petrea, 1951–.
Sometimes hearts have to break: 25 inspirational
journeys to healing and peace.

ISBN 978 1 74051 333 3.
ISBN 1 74051 333 9.

1. Terminally ill – Psychological aspects.
2. Terminally ill – Biography. I. Title.

362.19

Cover image by Louise Lister
Cover design by Nanette Backhouse, saso content & design pty ltd
Internal design based on that by Yolande Gray
Typeset by Midland Typesetters, Maryborough, Victoria
Printed and bound by Griffin Press

For Wendie who is a blessing in my life

CONTENTS

ACKNOWLEDGEMENTS

The people who have shared their stories with me deserve great appreciation and thanks. Without them this book would amount to nothing. Their names have been changed where requested or to protect the identity of those who courageously shared so much of themselves.

My partner Wendie patiently reassured me in dark moments that the book *was* worth writing and I thank her for her love and support. My family and friends also extended their love, feedback and constant encouragement – thank you.

The volunteers who attend our residential programs live the message of this book and make it possible for me to continue my work. My special thanks to Jenny Maher, Anne Stephen, Gillian Maxwell, Poppy Becher and Margaret Hahn, whose love and support is a constant source of joy to me.

My editor, Julia Stiles, has contributed much both in her skills as an editor and her encouragement to go deeper still. Thank you.

INTRODUCTION

Over the years I have often been asked why I work with people who are dying. Surely I must find it very depressing. Even hopeless at times.

This book is my answer. The following stories are full of hope – hope for the future, for healing, for finding peace in our lives, for reconciliation with the past. They are a tribute to the human spirit.

Since my recovery from leukaemia in 1984 I have counselled tens of thousands of people with life-threatening illnesses and facilitated thousands of support groups. In addition I've facilitated scores of residential programs for people with cancer, AIDS and other life-threatening illnesses, and taught many health professionals how to have a healthy relationship with their patients, how to avoid burnout, how to integrate natural therapies into oncology and palliative care, and how to facilitate effective support groups. This book comes out of those years of my own illness and recovery, and my witnessing of other people's struggles with a life-threatening illness and their search for peace and purpose in their lives. I wanted to show the joy and the pain; the sorrow and the happiness; the peace and the despair, so that we might all – well or sick – come to understand more fully the meaning and value of our lives.

To tell the stories of so many others without telling my own seemed to ignore a fundamental premise which I believe is invaluable in counselling. That is, the level to which I am willing to experience my own pain, fear, despair, love, joy or any other emotion, is the level to which I will be able to join with another in their own explorations. For instance, young parents who want to tell me of the awful anguish they feel about dying and the prospect of leaving their young children. I too have ventured into that dark chasm of fear and am willing to enter it again in the hope that by sharing the journey we can help each other shed a light upon the path. If I feel awkward and don't know what to say or do, then rest assured I will change the conversation through my body language, questions or responses.

My life has been blessed by many ups and downs. These experiences have pushed me to explore parts of myself I would otherwise never have willingly ventured into. My path to peace has led right through the heart of anguish. In telling my story I know that we will find common ground because our stories are all woven from a common thread. The events may differ but the paths are similar.

Life is full of uncertainties. It presents us with the unexpected, the unasked for and, sometimes, the unthinkable. We struggle to understand and accept these events, to find meaning in them. The quiet heroes of these stories have found resolution, humour, wisdom and much more through the unexpected events of their lives. Their stories show us all that the healing of our hearts is not only possible but that out of our suffering can come the precious gift of peace. By peace I don't mean a wishy-washy attitude of passive acceptance. I mean a dynamic state of being in which we feel that we can play an active part in our own healing process; a stare in which we feel passionate about living, find our challenges stimulating and satisfying, and feel deeply loved and supported by those in our lives.

Common sense tells us that someone who feels out of control of their lives and ambivalent about living, who feels that their challenges are overwhelming and that they aren't loved by anyone nor do they belong anywhere is unlikely to experience a deep sense of peace.

I don't know any dying people. I believe we're either alive or we're dead. Whilst we're alive we need the love, honour and respect due to any living person. These friends of mine that I will tell you about shortly are truly alive as they embrace each day, living it to its fullest potential. However, in order to find and fulfil life's potential, we must sometimes venture into the dark chasms of emotional, psychological and spiritual pain.

It took me many years to learn to acknowledge this pain. I never cried. I thought it was a sign of weakness.

Besides, I had such a backlog of unshed tears I was afraid that if I allowed myself to weep, I would never stop, and, worse still, I would disintegrate into a million fragments and never reintegrate. I was terrified I would fall into a black hole and never be able to climb out.

However, through the grace of my illness and in working with others confronting their own suffering, I stumbled upon a wonderful truth. It is OK to let our hearts break, because eventually they heal. In fact, as our hearts heal they increase our capacity for love. Because of the scar tissue, I suspect.

These days my eyes are often misty, but there's no longer a backlog of uncried tears. My eyes mist up when I'm touched by another's struggle; they mist up when my heart is full, when my eyes drink in beauty, when my heart soars with music or the sound of crickets and frogs in the night. They mist up when I'm immersed in being fully alive and present to the grand mystery of life. And, during counselling, when I join deeply with another and we experience that moment of connection in which we both feel heard and understood and our spirits feel nourished by one another. These are the sacred moments in a lifetime.

Most of us seem to think that we're meant to have blissful childhoods and happy teen years; enter the career of our choice and excel; find the perfect partner who loves, honours and respects us at all times; have children who obey and revere us; find our dream home and pay it off effortlessly; and then, when all that's done, go fishing in our old age. I'm not having one of those lives and I haven't met anyone else who is either!

We would be better served by understanding that life is a roller-coaster ride and that we can never be sure what lies over the crest or around the corner. That it is our responsibility to find and fasten our own 'seat belt' so that when the roller-coaster swings to the left when we could have sworn it was meant to go to the right, we're in a position to say: 'Ah! The scenery isn't quite what I expected, but this is what has happened, what am I going to do about it?'

Our seat belt can be any activity, belief or philosophy that promotes self-understanding and connects us deeply to our inner selves. For some this might be listening to music or being in nature; for others it might be religious, philosophical or spiritual beliefs, values or practices. Or it might be the company of good friends. Whatever connects us to our own inner knowledge of the truth about ourselves: this is what we must practise. Then we can experience life in all its varying colours as an opportunity for self-realisation.

If we don't have a seat belt, when the roller-coaster unexpectedly swings the 'wrong' way, we can easily get stuck with: 'Why me? It's not fair! I don't deserve this. It shouldn't have happened to me.' Feeling like that is healthy and understandable. I've never met anyone who deserves to have cancer or any other life-threatening illness. However, getting stuck with those feelings and not being able to move beyond them isn't the way to find peace and resolution. Finding resolution is essential because only then can painful events become part of our history rather than something that continues to dominate the present moment. Then, as we move forward on our journey, we can call upon the wisdom gleaned from the experience whenever we need to.

We cannot always control what happens to us, but we can play an active part in how we respond to what happens. To rail at life is to miss the opportunity for inner exploration and revelation. Life is not a competition to see who can stay alive the longest. What is important is not the length of our lives but the spirit and passion with which we live them.

The seat belt I have found most effective for myself and for gravely ill people is meditation, particularly group meditation. A special sort of energy is generated and all who participate, including the teacher, are strengthened. The group becomes a touchstone of peace at a time when spirits might be flagging or emotions chaotic.

Support groups are quite common now and they can be invaluable forums for people to tell their stories. The support groups I, and others trained by me, have held for many years at the Quest for Life Centre are somewhat different from other groups, however. They very deliberately, through their carefully developed structure and guidelines, create a safe, non-judgemental and accepting atmosphere in which each person feels valued and important.

Our groups enable people to tell their stories truthfully, without having to protect anyone from their suffering. Participants can feel safe to share without being told how to think or feel or what to do. Past traumas can be resolved so people can more fully participate in the present without the burden of the past.

It's true that each of us holds our own best answers within ourselves, but sometimes we need a safe environment in which to talk through our situation and so discover what those answers might be. Sometimes we don't know what we feel until we hear what we say. Family members are often so preoccupied with their own distress that they find it difficult to let loved ones explore their fears and concerns with them. If gravely ill people choose to confront their fears with those they love, they're often told to cheer up and be positive. However, being positive is being real with what's going on. For instance, it's far more positive to say, 'I feel frightened and confused and I hope tomorrow's a better day' than to say through gritted teeth that everything's fine when it's not.

People come to our support groups for many different reasons. To share their stories, to find companionship with people who have similar experiences, to learn from one another, to give support. All the people who come to share their stories inspire me and are my heroes. The mere presence of someone too terrified, distressed or anxious to talk touches me deeply and I am amazed at their courage to come to a group at all. Each one, even if they don't have a dramatic story to tell, has a story nonetheless. And each one has enriched my life and contributed to my being able to continue my work.

I sometimes use the following metaphor to explain the relationship between myself and those with whom I work. I think of myself as the guard of a railway station. Trains keep coming into the station and people get on and off. My job is to keep the station clean and tidy, the drink machine full and the rubbish bins empty. Then I can be free to sit a while and talk with those who wait at the station until they're ready to board another train. We share experiences, perceptions, laughter and the wisdom we have gathered from our journey thus far. We can sort through our baggage together and see if we're ready to discard anything superfluous; then we can repack with greater awareness those things which we value for the journey ahead or are not yet ready to discard. We can love each other unconditionally without any need to change or judge one another.

Some faces are just a blur as their train flashes by, and our contact is brief. Some come for a short time; others have stayed many years. When it is time for their departure we bid each other a warm farewell with shared blessings for both our journeys and gratitude in our hearts for having known one another. I remember each person more with the joy of having known them than with the sadness of their departure.

If I thought my job was to stop people from getting on or off the train, I'd be a wreck. My hope is that I've provided a little refreshment along the way and, if invited, shed a little light on the baggage travellers carry with them on their journey.

Although it is often because of crisis, illness or tragedy that we begin to seek real and deep healing, each of us has our own challenges to peace. We all benefit by finding peace within ourselves; in fact, the whole planet benefits. When we truly find wholeness, resolution and peace within ourselves we can become dynamic contributors to our friends, our families, our communities and our planet. We don't have to wait for a crisis to precipitate that healing process. Peace is definitely possible. We can choose to embark upon the journey of that healing simply because life can be so much richer as a result. Waiting for the excuse of illness or tragedy to set in motion that spiritual journey is only to postpone peace.

Finding a safe place in which to tell our story and have it deeply heard by someone who will not try to fix the problem is tremendously important. When a friend tells us about a problem, how often do we want to rush in to solve it? When our friend has a problem which can't be fixed, how do we deal with our own discomfort of not having the solution? It is often those who have experienced their own suffering that we turn to when we are faced with ours. These are companions of our heart who respect us enough to listen deeply to our story without offering any quick-fix solutions. They might ask questions or offer insights which can help us discover our individual strengths, but ultimately we must find our own solutions. Hearing their stories can provide us with ideas and the hope that we will eventually find our way, but each of us must find our own path to healing.

Every person I have worked with has brought me something of real value. Sometimes when I've been tired and emotionally drained they have stiffened my resolve, opened my heart yet again and restored my confidence in my ability to accompany them through their own maze of confusion or conflict.

They have made me even more aware of the depth of the human spirit in suffering, as well as the heights that come through the joy of sharing ourselves honestly.

I'd like to be on my deathbed fifty years from now and be able to say: 'That was a ripper. It was a good life, well lived.' In order to utter the blessing of those words, one must fully embrace life and be present to its mystery.

Let me first tell you my story, then I will introduce you to some friends who have shared in that blessing.

MY STORY

Ever since I arrived on this planet I've been trying to unravel the mysteries of life, to understand why we are here. As a child I didn't find a lot of answers to the mysteries, or support for my questioning.

I was the youngest of three children and much of my childhood was spent in trying to keep up with my two brothers, a task at which I never felt I succeeded. I was born eighteen months after my brother Brenden. He was an immensely talented and lovable person who absorbed most of the energy within our family until he took his own life when he was thirty-two. I worshipped the ground he walked on; in my eyes he could do no wrong. I took pride in being Brenden's sister and always sought his approval, which I never felt I received. This was probably a misconception born of the fact that my need for his approval was so great that it could never really be satisfied.

When my mother was nursing me as a baby, she would read or play with Brenden at the same time, otherwise he would be off setting fire to the house or causing some other such mischief. When she wasn't feeding me or attending to my other needs, Brenden would wrap his arms and legs around her waist and neck and hang onto her whilst she went about her day. I grew up thinking: 'Shh, be quiet. Brenden is really important.'

Such was the power of this ingrained message that when I was raped by a 'friend' at seventeen, my only reaction was to feel: 'Shh, be quiet. His needs are more important than mine. It'll be over soon.' It was my first sexual experience.

What made it worse was that there were people in the house who would have come had I screamed. The person who raped me had no gun and no knife, only determination and physical strength, and I was helpless against him. I dared not call out and could not even speak of it until I was in my mid-twenties. Even then I felt guilty, as if I must have deserved it because I had neither resisted nor called for help. But I'm jumping ahead of my story.

We lived in middle-class suburbia. There was no physical, sexual or emotional abuse; no divorce, nor threat of it. We looked like a happy family. Yet I always had a sense of impending disaster. There seemed to be a constant air of tension at home because of the potential within Brenden for emotional implosion. I found this very frightening, although no-one spoke of it, and it felt as though an invisible presence dominated my waking moments. Walking on emotional eggshells became my way of life.

As a young child I had experiences for which I could find no explanation. My language wasn't yet developed enough for me to articulate my questions, and even if it had been, I wouldn't have known how or whom to ask. One of these experiences happened when I was about seven years old.

It was a warm spring morning and I was playing in our front garden with our dog when suddenly the world around me became transparent. I could see through the earth, trees, plants, cars, horses and even Brynner, our dog.

Inside everything there was a glorious light which illuminated from within. It was like suddenly seeing the hand within the glove. I knew that light was within me and within all things, and that there was nothing in creation that did not have it as its cause. It was more substantial than bricks and mortar and it had no beginning nor ending. I knew it was the essence of all things. The light itself was indescribable. I cannot say how long I stood transfixed nor what I did immediately after. I do remember feeling that it was far more real than anything I'd experienced thus far in my life. It heightened my awareness of the presence of mystery and left me with an aching yearning to return to that state in which I had felt so intensely alive and at one with all things. It served as a beacon for many years.

Feeling that some of my wonderings were vaguely touched upon at church, I resolved to ask our minister some of my more perplexing questions. One sunny

Sunday morning after the family service, I summoned the courage to speak to him. In my child's mind this cassocked 'wise' man looming above me was an all-knowing authority. He stooped down to hear me ask 'What is beyond the stars?' He stood up, smiled and, without hesitation, told me that God had placed all the stars in the heavens within a huge egg.

I was puzzled, but undaunted; I continued by asking him how Adam and Eve had *really* got here. Again he replied that God had placed them inside an egg. I asked how they got out of the egg and he told me that God had given them a hammer and chisel.

I was shattered. I felt belittled and embarrassed and was certain that I had stumbled upon a conspiracy in which I was never to be told the truth. The minister had not only lied to me but had exposed me as someone unworthy to utter even the questions. I retreated further into my inner world and my sense of isolation grew.

Brenden and I knew that we had what we referred to as 'black holes' within us, a darkness which could not be talked about and therefore couldn't be resolved. I felt very much as though I'd landed on the wrong planet and, though I did my best to learn the language and the ways of the inhabitants, I would never belong. I ached for contact with people from my own planet. Years later I, like many others, became a blubbering heap when I saw the movie *ET.* Seeing ET distraught and pointing to the heavens saying 'Home' always brought me undone.

These feelings Brenden and I shared may not have stemmed from the same cause, and I don't remember that we ever consciously named them, but we shared a knowledge of something awful that lurked within us. It terrorised us, each in our own ways. Brenden's torment with depression and despair always seemed worse than mine and I tried hard not to have any needs because Brenden's were more than enough for any one household.

For me this led to a dislocation between who I presented to the world and who I was to myself. I felt tormented because I was so afraid of not getting it right, of not measuring up to some self-imposed standard. I thought there must be something wrong with me because, other than Brenden, no-one else seemed to have these struggles. For instance, if I achieved ninety-five per cent in a music exam, I could only see that I'd made five mistakes. This pressure was never exerted upon me by my parents. Perhaps it came instead from a 'fire and brimstone' minister we had at our church. He told us that to think a bad thought was as bad as putting that thought into action. He also told us that non-Christians would burn forever, gnashing their teeth in a place of torment. As a child I seemed to take much of what I heard very literally. I would wake at night grinding my teeth and would take it as an indication that I was destined for damnation. I felt completely inadequate and was loathe to grow into puberty because of the added pressures I knew people had to face as they matured. This inner reality was reflected in my small stature. Most of my peers were sprouting breasts, periods and boyfriends, whilst my body was still that of a child.

Just after my twelfth birthday I suddenly grew nine

inches in one year. This took me from being a very small child to an average sized one. This rapid growth caused an imbalance between muscle and bone growth and I developed painful calluses under both my feet as the bones in my legs grew crookedly and my knees rotated inwards. My knees became swollen and painful and walking became all but impossible.

After months of intense but unsuccessful physiotherapy, I entered hospital for the first of several major orthopaedic operations to straighten my bones so that I could walk again.

This surgery involved years of plaster casts, callipers, traction, crutches, walking sticks, physiotherapy and the tedium of learning to walk all over again. It also ended my school days, something for which I was grateful as school had never been a place of joy for me. However, even correspondence lessons soon became difficult because of the frequency with which I had general anaesthetics.

In hospital I felt confined and safe for the first time in my life. I escaped school, where I was miserable, and living with Brenden, whom I adored but found painful, scary and a challenge to be around. I became immersed in a world of adults, a world in which I felt much happier. I received unending love and support from my mother who visited every day, even though she was stretched thin by a new business venture and worrying about Brenden who was entering into the real beginnings of his crippling depression.

I was in traction for nine months during this time because my femur would not unite. In an effort to straighten my leg the surgeons had cut through the femur and rotated my lower leg outwards by eleven degrees and then plated it into place. I never left my bed during those long months and, needless to say, had to attend to all bodily functions in the confines of the bed. I found performing on a bedpan completely impossible if there was so much as a crack in the curtains. Yet I was far too shy to ask anyone to make any necessary adjustments. I resolved this dilemma by eating as little as possible so I wouldn't need the bedpan as often. I grew thinner and my bones struggled to find the nutrients necessary for healing.

I entered my teen years full of trepidation. I didn't feel I had the emotional stamina to play the games in which I saw others take a seeming pleasure. Pain and discomfort were realities I could trust, and to some extent control, and my outer world virtually shrank to the confines of my hospital bed.

I developed terrible cramps in the wasted muscles of my legs, which frequently ended in my passing out. First my toes would curl over, then the arch of my foot, then the calf and thigh muscles and on into my hip. Because one leg was in traction and the other in plaster, I couldn't move to relieve the inexorable cramping within the muscles. Medication didn't alleviate the agony and my eyes became lined with wrinkles.

One day an elderly woman came to visit me. To this day neither my parents nor I know who she was. Perhaps she was an angel or some figment of my imagination, but either way she gave me a great gift. She wore a hat and gloves and carried a handbag over her arm, and she looked like everyone's image of a granny. She seemed to know everything about me and the pain I was experiencing. She told me that when I next felt a cramp coming on, I should take a deep breath and go to a quiet place inside myself where I could watch the pain.

I found this an intriguing idea. The first and each subsequent time that I practised this, I found myself looking down on my body from the ceiling. I could see my body going through the motions of cramping, and I was aware of the strong sensation of the contracting muscles, yet there was no pain attached to it.

This means of escape was a real blessing. In addition I was kept on morphine for a long time after each operation. Morphine and being able to escape to the ceiling were my two main mechanisms for coping with the pain.

Eventually my doctor told me there was a strong possibility that my femur would not unite and that it was time to consider a wheelchair. This provided a great impetus for me to get up and walk! Even school looked terrific by comparison.

Each night, between nurses' rounds, as quietly as I could, I'd disconnect the weights that hung from the end of my right leg. I'd let them squeak, squeak, squeak their way down to the floor. My legs were like pencils lying inertly in the bed. I could circle my calf with my thumb and third finger. Mustering every ounce of willpower, I still could not move them. They were ugly, hairy, unwelcome strangers sharing my bed, and, even worse, they were attached to me. Each night I would drag myself out of the sheets and, supporting myself on my elbows, attempt to struggle around the bed. For the first two or three nights my bones grated unbearably as I tried to put weight upon the unhealed leg.

However, much to everyone's surprise and delight, within three weeks the bones in my leg had united. I had unknowingly dislodged the plate and screws holding the bones together, but once these were surgically removed, my leg continued to heal and physiotherapy began once again. I never told a soul about my nightly escapades, though they must have wondered how the plates and screws had become displaced.

Between the surgeries to my legs I was allowed to leave hospital and I would be sent to the country to my god-mother's home to recuperate. Their household contained only adults and I loved the stories of the land they shared over meals around the dining table. They would drag out encyclopaedias and dictionaries to clarify or explore some topic under discussion. My godmother's sister-in-law, Madge, was a wise woman of the land who could pick up a clod of dirt, smell it and tell me what was missing from the soil and how long since it had rained. Madge knew all the birds and would call to them in the trees as we walked or rode, and she could tell the movements of the animals by their tracks. I was a hungry sponge ready to soak up information and I revelled in the freedom I felt in the country.

I'd often make my way on crutches to the paddock above the house and watch the closing of the day. A certain stillness would descend as the colours changed from the harsh brightness of daylight to the softening shades of dusk. The chooks, prompted by some internal clock, retreated to their night shelter; the sheep filed with purposeful tread towards higher ground; the geese by the creek ceased their cackling as they settled for the night; cows collected and suckled their calves; birds chattered to one another, organising their sleeping places. Effie, the old housekeeper, would limp her way to secure the dogs to their chains, handing them titbits from the kitchen and talking to them softly. The plum-coloured hills slowly melted into darkness and the evening star would twinkle in the heavens as it heralded the coming night's display of grandeur. This scene worked some magic within my soul and brought me comfort. I felt at once completely insignificant in the grand scheme of things and yet at the centre of my own universe. It was as if nothing else existed outside this moment. Perhaps the nearby town of Merriwa did not exist because I could not perceive it. Perhaps nothing existed other than my own perception.

Each time I returned to the city I would ache for the country and its solitude. Nature had her rhythms and cycles and went about her business with certainty. There wasn't much that was tentative in nature. Everything moved towards its blossoming and fulfilment and seemed to do so with enthusiasm.

When I was finally free of callipers and plasters and my legs were strong enough for me to spend some time in the saddle, I rode about the paddocks assisting cows who needed help calving. It was the mid-sixties and there was a drought on. The cows were so poorly nourished that they had little energy to expel their calves, or the misshapen bodies of their young made giving birth impossible. I would reach deep inside the cow, reassuring her – and myself – by crooning softly as I felt for the legs of her calf and hauled it safely into the world. I wondered what kind of a world I was dragging this small animal into and whether it would have the necessary spirit to survive against such bitter odds.

Back in the city I wrote agonised letters to my godmother about the meaninglessness of life there. Why were people cooped up in little boxes piled one upon another? Why did they spend their days shuffling paper from one side of a desk to the other? What was the purpose of it all? Was this the way we were meant to blossom and fulfil our destiny, or was it only nature who moved with certainty along prescribed lines? What was wrong with me that I couldn't settle for life in the way that I saw most of my peers doing?

At seventeen I began nursing but resigned after a year. I couldn't use my knees adequately to lift patients and the strain on my lower back was too much. The call of the country was ever present and I explored a range of occupations, including roustabouting in New Zealand shearing sheds and boundary riding in western Queensland.

When I became fed up with the formality of life in the homestead, I would work outside as a boundary rider, mending fences after kangaroos, emus or wild pigs had broken through them. At night I would sleep on the earth under a canopy of stars. It was a time of solitude and contemplation and it was during this time that I learned to meditate.

I would get up at about five every morning and work

until nine. By then it was too hot to work as the temperature would often soar into the high forties. I would make a little canvas shelter over a bore drain, which provided the sheep and cattle with water from deep artesian wells, and sit in the water all day until around five in the afternoon when it was cool enough to emerge. I'd continue working until about ten o'clock at night, then crawl into my swag and, gazing up into the heavens, drift off into a contented sleep. Sitting in the bore drain I would read esoteric, philosophical and spiritual books written by some of the world's great thinkers and, out of their collected wisdom, I taught myself to meditate. The peace and stillness of the bush was a beautiful backdrop to meditation and I found joy in the richness of each moment. I would also use it as a way of escaping the questions which still lurked within my mind. Why were we here and for what purpose? Was there absolute meaning or only the one I ascribed to the events of a lifetime?

At night the heavens were a stage upon which the mystery of the planets and their rotation was played out for my isolated observation. Lying in my swag under the open sky I could witness the almost imperceptible movement of our planet in relation to the heavens as stars rose and set. Shooting stars were always magical and the excitement of witnessing them never dimmed for me.

I was often awestruck by the beauty of my surroundings and the wonder of nature. My first reaction to the landscape of western Queensland was that the countryside was empty and dead. But as I lived with the land's rhythms and cycles I began to see its richness and beauty and to know the many creatures who shared this habitat in which I was a mere fragile and vulnerable guest.

The life of a roustabout or a boundary rider is demanding for anyone and I made no allowances for my physical limitations. I treated my legs almost as if they were my enemy; if they faltered, it only made me drive myself harder. Riding a horse was probably the most demanding and destructive physical activity for anyone with my surgical history. But physical pain was one touchstone of reality that I could rely on. I felt ill equipped to give any expression to all the feelings which fermented within me and this somehow put me at war with my own body.

When I was nineteen I had further surgery to straighten my right leg. Since then I've needed several arthroscopic procedures to clean out the cavity within the knee, and five years ago I had another major operation to stop the same leg from bowing. However, I am fortunate to have such good use of my legs considering both my surgical history and my abuse of them.

Back in the city I became increasingly disabled by osteoarthritic pain in my knees so I began to refine my diet more and more stringently. During my childhood I had opted for vegetarianism several times. The choice then was more about not wanting to be responsible for the death of animals, but my mother would cook the most delicious roast and I would succumb to the wonderful smell of roast lamb and mint peas. Later this choice was based both on my philosophical viewpoint and on a belief that meat was not only unnecessary for our health and wellbeing but might also be detrimental. I cut out tea, coffee and alcohol. I ate no red or white meats, no cheese or other dairy products. Gradually the arthritis improved, though that may have been as much from becoming less demanding of my legs as from dietary changes.

However, for all my interest in diet and the changes I made, there were certainly some anomalies. The questions of existence still preoccupied me and my search led me in the direction of illegal drugs. In 1972 I travelled to Amsterdam, the European capital of the hippy boom and a place where drugs were freely available.

My brothers had been travelling around Asia and Europe for some time and Brenden had been living in Holland for a couple of months. He had escaped the grasp of the psychiatrists back home who seemed only to drug him into senselessness. He'd undergone months of hospitalisation, electric-shock therapy, endless group psychotherapy, and drugs which reduced him to a zombie. He wanted to deal with his inner torment in his own way and for that he had my support. We settled into a singularly bohemian lifestyle on a boat on one of Amsterdam's canals.

The atmosphere in the city at the time was enormously exciting. People were wearing flowers in their hair and sleeping in the Vondel Park in the centre of Amsterdam. We questioned the authority of the Church, the government, modern medicine, the philosophy of the western economy and the traditions of our culture. I enjoyed marijuana and hashish and very soon started to use LSD on an almost daily basis.

The first time I took LSD was a similar experience to the many times I had had morphine in the past. I liked the changed reality these drugs produced. They gave me new and diverse perceptions about the questions that had long tormented me.

However, after several months of taking LSD I couldn't function properly at all. I could barely talk and had to be told when to eat and go to bed and so on. I couldn't bear to be confined in small places and frequently experienced panic attacks about almost anything.

I had moved to a farm in the southern province of Zeeland in Holland. After several months in this state of fear and confusion, I had an experience which, by grace, was to be the catalyst for change and healing.

I have always been an early riser. Each day, before everyone else on the farm was up, I'd sweep the lounge room, put fresh water in the flower bowls, empty the incense holders and plump up the cushions. On this particular morning, I had attended to my chores and was listening to Vivaldi's *Four Seasons* when suddenly a shaft of sunlight broke through the grey Dutch sky and illuminated a bowl of bright yellow chrysanthemums on the table in front of me.

I was struck by the beauty of this and heard, as clearly as if a voice had sounded in my ear: 'If you don't leave the farm within the hour and Holland today, you will lose all power of discrimination.' Such was the magnitude of this moment that I immediately packed my belongings into a plastic bag, hitchhiked to Amsterdam and flew to England, arriving at Heathrow that same day with precisely ten pounds in my pocket.

I only knew one person in London whom I felt I could contact at that time but had no idea where to find her. I travelled into Piccadilly and was sitting in a coffee shop when, amongst the twelve million people in London that summer, my one friend, Hagit, walked past. She was from Israel and I had met her only briefly at a youth hostel in Holland at the beginning of my stay there. She was returning to Israel almost immediately.

I stayed with Hagit for two days during which time I went to Australia House and, to my own astonishment, got a job as a nanny in the Sussex countryside. My ability to pass myself off as an ordinary person was somewhat hindered by my strange hobbling gait, my lack of suitable clothes and my fear of social contact. Being in the English countryside in the company of small children proved to be a time of great healing for me and I gradually began to be more at ease amongst people.

When I returned to Australia I embarked once more upon my nursing studies. I was continually struck by how well modern medicine helped people with acute illnesses, yet seemed at a loss when dealing with any chronic or degenerative diseases. I felt as though we were always mopping up after the milk had been spilt. We had excellent mops but I became increasingly interested in what might be needed to create a more stable, less susceptible glass.

Death and dying were subjects only just beginning to be spoken of when I was nursing. In the last hours of a patient's life we would usually draw the curtains around them and from time to time a nurse would peep behind the curtains and whisper to us that they were still breathing. Once someone was dead, we would respectfully wash and attend to the body and deliver it to the morgue.

Many of my colleagues thought me strange because I sought out the patients who were close to death. I could feel their aloneness, and their noises, smells and behaviour weren't frightening to me. It felt a privilege to be with them. By holding their hand, reading to them or even singing quietly – so that none of the other nurses would hear – I created a sense of reassurance for myself as well as the patient. This might be a lonesome journey for them, but I would be there to watch over them and accompany them to the 'door'. We would watch and wait together.

Our nursing instructor had told us that hearing was the last of our faculties to go and that we needed to be very aware of this as we ministered to a patient's needs. This had made a big impact on me because of an incident when I was fifteen. One of Brenden's friends had been involved in a motorcycle accident and was unconscious for several months. I had visited him in the head injuries unit of Royal North Shore Hospital. I'd taken Robbie's hand and asked him to squeeze it if he could hear me. Within a couple of moments he had done so and that proved to be the beginning of his long but complete recovery. My speaking to Robbie had caused quite a stir amongst the staff in his ward because, at that time, it was believed that unconscious patients were beyond the reach of words. So later, during my training, I had taken very much to heart what we'd been told about patients who appear to be unresponsive.

Mrs O'Sullivan was a patient who taught me much about being good company to those who appeared to be beyond words. She had been involved in a car accident and had not regained consciousness. It was now many months later and though she looked as if she was sleeping peacefully, it was the sleep of unconsciousness. I was on night duty when Mrs O'Sullivan was assigned to me. Each morning I'd walk into her room to wash her and to change the linen on her bed. Whilst I was doing this I would talk about the dawn sky or my plans for the day or some other titbit of information from my life. I always spoke her name and treated her with care and respect. From my ramblings she probably knew more about me than any of my colleagues and it's a wonder that she didn't die of boredom then and there!

After each stint of night duty I would have four days off. Imagine my surprise and delight on returning to work one day to find that Mrs O'Sullivan had regained consciousness.

The moment I walked into her room and greeted her, her eyes flew open and she grabbed my hand. What she told me has stayed with me ever since. She spoke of her anger and frustration at the doctors on their rounds when they would stand at the bottom of her bed and say they didn't expect her ever to regain consciousness. She felt they glossed over her as if she were already dead. She had wanted to scream at them that she was very much alive and a force to be reckoned with. She spoke of the language of touch – often she had been handled roughly or carelessly because the nurse didn't think she was 'there'. And she spoke with gratitude of the inane chatter I used to inflict on her each day. She called it her lifeline.

One particular event involving an eighty-two-year-old woman with leukaemia proved to be the last straw in my nursing career. Evy had no family and I never once saw her have a visitor during the weeks she was in our ward. She was not undergoing any further treatment and we knew this would be her last admission. I had only been assigned to look after her on a couple of occasions. She was a very quiet and dignified woman and most of her days were spent dozing.

Evy died one afternoon whilst I was on duty. To my horror and astonishment a code blue alert was sounded and her cubicle became a hive of activity. The young doctors injected her with heart-stimulating drugs and used the shock of electrical currents to remind her heart of its once effortless function.

I was utterly dismayed. Why couldn't she be left in her dignified peace? Why did we rail against death? Where was the respect due her? I was so upset I made an appointment with the director of nursing to discuss my concerns. She listened patiently but then said bluntly, 'They have to practise on somebody.'

I could not believe that this was sufficient a reason for such invasive action. Surely the moment of our death could be made sacred by those who were privileged to be by our side. I would have felt differently had the hospital gained Evy's permission to practise upon her after her death. Instead, she was helpless against their abuse.

Disheartened, I left nursing a second time and began to study naturopathy. I was interested in the relationship between why we get ill and how we get well, and what place illness plays in our lives. The naturopathic course provided a lot of clues and many practical skills, but ultimately I didn't feel it was the whole answer to these questions.

It was during the time of my studies that I met and married Leo. We shared many interests including those of health, philosophy, the world's religions, and purpose and meaning in our lives. Leo has an infectious enthusiasm and joy about life and from these qualities I drew both strength and comfort. Not long after we married, our daughter Kate was born and almost four years later our son Simon completed our family. In their first few years I studied part-time and was able to devote myself to their care. Young children live so wholeheartedly in the present moment and I found joy in watching them explore their world and develop into loving little people. Living in suburbia with babies had never appealed to me – I had always thought I'd be off exploring the Amazon or some such thing – and yet this time of nurturing Kate and Simon was a precious oasis in which the child within me was also nourished.

Not long after I had finished my naturopathic studies, Brenden took his life in Kathmandu. He'd struggled with depression since his teen years and had been hospitalised, therapised, worried over, encouraged and supported – all to no avail. He called our mother his 'never-give-up mum'. On several occasions he'd been rushed to hospital in time to have his stomach pumped, and we all knew he ached deeply for normality and to be content with a world he could only see as on a path to disaster.

He had told me when we were not even out of primary school that he knew he had to take his own life by the time he was thirty. Instead, he found Muktananda, an Indian spiritual teacher, at thirty and his life began to change for the better. He no longer struggled with depression and meditation finally became something he could draw deeply upon and gain peace from. For two years he seemed to have found a stability and contentment none of us had ever dreamed possible, and we were immensely relieved and grateful for this miracle. This peace that Brenden had found made the shock of his death even more powerful.

Brenden travelled to India and entered an ashram in order to be closer to Muktananda. The whole family breathed a sigh of relief as we contemplated life without the continuous worry over Brenden. Then, without warning, we received a phone call from the Department of Foreign Affairs saying he was dead. His body was cremated by a river in Kathmandu. We held neither funeral nor memorial service – our grieving was a private affair – and continued with our lives, though the aching grief continued also.

Brenden had always lived in a world apart from ours. As the news of his death filtered through the grapevines that connected to the worlds we could not access, we began to receive letters and calls from strangers. He was enormously loved by more people than most, and many of his friends were the 'night people' for whom the knowledge of his death brought great pain and the reminder of life's fragility. Yet even so they called us to share in our sadness. We heard stories of Brenden's 'other' life, of him helping this person get off drugs or that person create a home for herself and her children. He had been a messenger of hope for others even though he had struggled to find any for himself.

It was difficult to grieve for someone who was in Kathmandu one moment and nowhere the next. There were none of the rituals of remembrance, no packing up of possessions, no tidying up of affairs. Some months later we received his wallet with one Australian dollar in it and a return airline ticket. We had precious few photos of him, one or two paintings and some letters. He created an aching presence when he was here and a greater aching void when he left.

Not long after Brenden's death, Leo and I and our two children moved to an ashram in America so that we could study yoga and meditation. The community of Ananda was nestled in the beautiful foothills of the Sierra Nevada mountains in northern California. It was one of the oldest spiritual communities in America and was founded on the teachings of Paramahansa Yogananda whose book, *Autobiography of a Yogi*, had been a guiding light to me.

Leo and I had long been struggling with our relationship. Though we still shared many interests, it was our devotion to our children and their future which had kept us together. The strain of Brenden's death became the catalyst for us to separate. Four weeks after our arrival at Ananda, Leo returned to Australia.

Some months later I graduated as a teacher of yoga and meditation. I grappled ever more deeply with the questions of human existence but found few satisfying answers. As I gained more knowledge through studying the Bhagavad-gita, the Upanishads, the Bible and Mahabharata, my life became split between a theoretical understanding of life and the lack of peace which continued to dominate my experience. My meditation practice was done as a twice-daily discipline but lacked heart and passion. I tried to live according to the truths I was studying, but the turbulence of my unresolved grief and questioning fermented just below the surface. I tried so hard to find peace and yet peace eluded me.

At the end of the course in yoga and meditation-teacher training I was invited to stay on as secretary and housekeeper to Swami Kriyananda who was the founder of the community where the course was held. It was during this time that I was diagnosed with acute myeloid leukaemia and my world fell apart. My prognosis was horrifying, and at the time of diagnosis the specialist told me I wouldn't be alive for Christmas – a mere twelve weeks away. The only treatment I was offered was chemotherapy which, he said, would neither put me into remission nor give me hope of a cure but would only extend my life by a few extra weeks. Had he painted a brighter picture about the advantages of chemotherapy I probably would have chosen it despite its cost and toxicity, two other factors which he emphasised. But I felt that I'd rather die 'healthy' of leukaemia than die feeling ravaged by chemotherapy. My mother flew to America to help me pack for my return to Australia.

My search for peace had led me through physical and emotional pain and suffering; through drug abuse, constant questioning, my brother's torment and death, my divorce, and then, at thirty-three, through single parenthood and now leukaemia. How could I have brought children into the world only to leave them? How could my parents possibly cope with my death on top of Brenden's? Was I to die before I found peace or any answers to the questions which had always tormented me?

I was born eighteen months after Brenden and, if I died on time, would be dead eighteen months after him.

I felt ambivalent about living. I was so tired of trying to get it right, to measure up to some impossible standard that I'd set myself, and I was weary of living with so much fear and grief. I'd been a strict vegetarian for fifteen years. I had completed a number of fasts of twenty, thirty and even forty days. I'd meditated regularly for fifteen years. I was trained as a naturopath, herbalist, homeopath, massage therapist and had finished my studies in yoga and meditation. To be diagnosed with leukemia was a slap in the face – I thought I had been doing everything right. My belief systems were shattered.

On my return I moved into my parents' home, whilst my children lived with their father. I was unable to care for them even on the weekends when they came to stay with me. The exhaustion was overwhelming and within a few short weeks I was virtually confined to my bed. Even showering and dressing became an ordeal and if I managed to shower myself, my mother would have to dry me. My hair came out in handfuls and it was depressing to see the long strands snaking their way across the shower recess floor and sliding down the drain. I felt like I was disintegrating before my very own eyes. I had not felt particularly sick at the time of my diagnosis but the rapidity of my deterioration was frightening.

Much as I was grateful for my mother's care I was also frustrated and depressed that I could no longer look after my needs nor those of my children. I was used to taking care of my own family and to move back into my parents' home and become a 'child' again in need of my mother's care was often a challenge in itself.

I gradually withdrew into a world of despair from which I thought I would never emerge. My parents would have done anything to support me and wanted to understand what I was thinking and feeling. However, despair is all consuming and to articulate such feelings generally requires distance from their intensity. Even if I had had a language to articulate my grief, I was loathe to further burden my parents when Brenden's death still loomed so large in all our hearts.

I had a deep mistrust of doctors and the medical system and was determined to avoid hospitals and being a patient ever again. If I was going to die then I wanted to conduct my end in my own way. The only doctor I was willing to consult with was our family GP, who for many years had also seen us through Brenden's traumas.

I got my will and financial affairs in order. My parents and I had some tentative and long overdue conversations about the past; I made tapes for my children and wrote them letters to be read in the future. Once these practical matters were attended to, I spent my days resting and began to meditate with a more open simplicity. I also had endless hours to think. I seesawed between feeling trapped by my powerlessness to change what was happening in my body and a sense of liberation as I let go in each moment of meditation. The contrast between these states of mind was extraordinary.

I would sit to meditate and into my mind would come the thought, 'What if I'm not here for Christmas?' Hot on its heels other thoughts would follow. 'How will my children cope? How will my parents cope? How will I cope? Who will come to the funeral? What will they say? Who'll be wearing my clothes in six months?' These thoughts would plague me and I could feel myself go down the emotional slippery slope to despair. It was obvious to me that most of my suffering was caused by my mind either leaping into the future or chewing over the past. But it was so difficult to keep my mind focused in the present when the thoughts that would lead to feelings of panic, despair or fear assailed me. Gradually I began to see that the same train of thoughts brought me undone each time and that they never served a useful purpose. They undermined my peace and made a mockery of my meditation. So I made an appointment with my worries, but when I sat at the appointed time to concentrate on them, none of them appeared. I came to see that the only power these worries had was when they snuck into my mind at unguarded moments. With this understanding and lots of practice, I was able to witness the 'What if I'm not here for Christmas?' thought and let it go.

Sometimes I was overwhelmed with the feeling that I hadn't *lived* yet. I had *done* many things in my life and my father could have gone on at length at my funeral about the diversity of my life's experiences. But *inside* I didn't feel like I'd really lived. That was more about a sense of personal peace and acceptance of who I was and the life I'd lived.

Once again I felt the incredible insignificance of my life in the grand scheme of things, whilst at the same time my life was terribly important to me. All the religious studies that I had embarked upon gave me little comfort. Life after death or reincarnation were of little significance to me for I was deeply attached to the people I loved and felt that my life had never amounted to more than the value of those relationships.

Lying in my bed, overlooking Sydney's Middle Harbour, these and other thoughts preoccupied my mind. The contrast between the beauty outside my room and the misery within my own head was not lost on me. Water sparkled in the sunlight; children played on the sand; tiny sailboats scudded across the harbour; soft clouds drifted through the blue heavens; leaves rustled in the breezes, and warm sunshine filled the room in which I sat untouched by the joy of life unfolding in front of me.

Paradoxically, the more I prepared to die the stronger

I seemed to become physically. The more I accepted life's fragility, the more I found strengths within myself. I felt I needed a time of isolation and solitude to explore more deeply this path to peace but was unsure of how to bring that about. My health evened out, though I was still weak and troubled by night sweats and bone pain.

My daughter Kate stood by my bed one day and said, 'Mum, you're sick. If you need to meditate to get well, then I think you should go back to Ananda.' Kate knew that meditation was the foundation upon which the community of Ananda was built and that I would have unlimited love and support from the people who were our friends there.

It was not an easy decision to make, but after discussions with my parents and reassurances to and from my children, I packed my life into a small suitcase and embarked once more for America. A few weeks after my arrival at Ananda, Swami Kriyananda was due to leave for Italy to lecture and he suggested that I accompany him and his entourage. On this occasion, instead of travelling around Europe, he was stationed in a villa near Lake Como in the north of Italy and people were to travel there for his teaching. Swami lectured fluently in four languages and the villa was filled with people from more than twenty-six countries.

My need for solitude was still strong but I was learning to trust that everything was unfolding in the manner that was right for me. I spent my days resting, practising yoga and meditation, and listening to Swami's lectures. The mountain air and the surrounding countryside were pristine and I sometimes ventured out for walks in the beautiful hills around the town of Veglio far above Lake Como.

At the conclusion of Swami's time in Italy I decided to devote myself more fully to meditation and so travelled to the beautiful town of Assisi which I had visited previously. I was unsure of where I would stay but I also sensed that it was time for the period of solitude I had been yearning for.

On the second afternoon of my visit I travelled the four and a half kilometres to the monastery known as the Hermitage. This monastery was built around a number of caves where Saint Francis and his close friends would go to meditate and pray. I stayed on after the tourists had left for the day and watched dusk settle over the beautiful plains of Perugia. I was joined by the *superiore* of the monastery, Father Ilarino. Though we shared no common language I felt an immediate bond with him. Through our halting attempts at communication he established that I was most welcome to stay in a little room kept for the purpose of solitary retreats. The following day I retrieved my belongings from the monastery where I had stayed in Assisi and moved into the Hermitage.

The Franciscan monks watched over me but allowed me solitude and space. Our lack of a common language meant that they never pried into my world, yet they must have wondered about this pale woman who took refuge in their monastery and in the cave Saint Francis had used for his meditations. They would make clucking noises over the photos of my children, pat me benevolently on the head and present me with a meal that was the antithesis of everything I had eaten in the past.

The first meal they presented to me contained meat and accompanying it was a goblet of wine and a chunk of white bread. I had eaten no meat, fish or chicken, nor drunk any alcohol, tea or coffee for fifteen years. I had been telling people during that time that 'the whiter the bread, the sooner you're dead!' Sitting at that ancient table I felt humbled by their loving care of me, a stranger. I had spent my life trying to get it right and here I was sick, on a mountain top in Italy away from my children and parents. I realised that I knew nothing. I ate whatever they presented to me with gratitude. It felt more important to surrender the rigid beliefs I had about diet and focus more on trusting that I was cared for and that I didn't have to earn my recovery.

In the first weeks of being in the cave for up to eighteen hours a day, I focused only on my shortcomings, my failings. I suspect I could still be sitting in that cave doing the same thing for the list seemed endless. The more I looked for faults, the more I found. I realised that I often used meditation techniques in a negative way to avoid confronting and resolving the hobgoblins which festered within me. But to acknowledge the full force of my despair, grief and fear seemed impossible. If fears or anxieties arose, I could use techniques of contemplation as a way of switching my awareness to something else. It was as if I was trying to put a layer of peace over my distress.

My relationships were up to date, I wrote daily postcards to my children. I often felt useless and unnecessary to the world. My children would cope, my parents would cope; surely it would be easier to let go and die. I felt like I knew how to do a good death, but I still didn't have a clue how to do a good life.

The only relief from my self-absorbed view of the world came through meditation, beautiful music or nature. Music expressed feelings and found resolution, neither of which I was able to do. Nature constantly sought to grow, blossom and return to itself only to repeat the process in another form.

As terrified as I was of the black hole within me, I knew that was where life and healing would be found. Not necessarily physical healing but that deeper healing wherein I could find a moment of peace. Although Brenden had plunged into his black hole never to emerge, I began to suspect that light and peace lay in close proximity to the darkness and that my journey wouldn't be complete until the darkness within myself was explored and addressed.

I felt I'd created an internal structure or scaffolding from which I could handle life. This internal scaffolding was made up of beliefs, attitudes and judgements and gave me the false sense of being able to remain in control of my life. I felt that in order to find peace and healing I'd have to let go this self-created and cherished structure. But it was the only way I knew how to live. To let go would require trust and I only had a very shaky willingness.

Most of us don't realise that we *do* have a choice in how we respond to each moment of our lives. If we don't realise this possibility then we simply react to situations. These reactions are borne out of our responses to our individual history. For instance, my response to Brenden's dominance in our household was to believe that I was less important. This entrenched belief meant that I would become 'powerless' in the face of many situations in my life, putting my needs below everyone else's. Had my response to Brenden's dominance been one of anger, perhaps my reactions later in life would have placed my needs *above* everyone else's.

Taking responsibility for the way I reacted to life meant that I could no longer blame anyone or anything for how I felt. I could rail at my childhood, the hospitalisations, rape, Brenden's depression and ultimate suicide, my marriage, separation and leukaemia, but whilst ever I railed I would exclude the possibility of peace. To accept these as the events of my life and to weep the long-held tears associated with them proved to be the path to peace.

There's nothing quite like being stuck between a rock and a hard place to help us to move forward. Finally I tiptoed to the door of despair and pushed it open. I went through an agonising yet liberating process of allowing and witnessing the despair I felt. Then came loneliness, grief, isolation, rejection and abandonment. Fear and panic, terror, anger and more despair. Feelings I had locked up for a lifetime came one by one or in groups that were impossible even to identify. I let myself feel them all. I wept buckets, railed at my powerlessness against what *is*, and surrendered my will to each moment as it unfolded.

It was in the cave where Saint Francis prayed that I learned more deeply that I couldn't necessarily change what was happening to me, but I could change the way I responded to it. These small discoveries were welcomed revelations and, in time, this led to a deep sense of peace and an acceptance of my future, regardless of the outcome of my disease.

When I got ready to die it was as if I had the whole of my life packed up into a little suitcase ready for an overseas trip and then the plane was cancelled.

The fact that I was still alive months after my diagnosis was as much a surprise to me as it was to everyone else. To this day I cannot be sure why I didn't die. I certainly don't feel I cured myself. That would be far too cheeky a thing to claim. For me the most miraculous part of my healing was that I had finally found a measure of peace which felt like a balm to the whole of my being. I wanted to experience that peace amongst those that I loved, in my work, in leisure and in every part of my life.

I found going into remission had its own particular challenges. The doctor said that I wasn't meant to have a remission and that it might only last a few weeks or, at most, months. I was faced with uncertainty. How much should I unpack the suitcase? Should I apply for a one-year or a ten-year driver's licence renewal? Should I get my teeth fixed? Was it worth buying a new pair of shoes when I might not get the wear out of them? Should I rent or buy? Should my children come back and live with me? All kinds of questions that most people don't ever think about suddenly became paramount. When you feel that the carpet has been well and truly pulled out from under your feet, it is difficult to feel any sense of security about life ever again. I was very careful about unpacking that suitcase.

Gradually I came to realise that we only have a moment to grow and blossom upon the earth and then we must leave. Even if we live to a hundred and six, it is all over and done with so quickly. We are not warming up for the big event; this isn't a dress rehearsal, it's the real thing. When we feel a deep preciousness about life it is a real blessing, and it is a blessing that we don't want to lose once we have discovered it.

Initially I lived very much as a tourist. And there's a lot to be said for living like that. To drink in every day as if it were both your first and your last. To savour moments rather than lose whole days through lack of awareness. In a way we are all tourists, embarked upon our own journey through life, and yet we so easily lose the sparkle of each moment as we become weighed down with careers, mortgages and other responsibilities.

My sense of uncertainty and the expectation that my remission was only temporary plagued my mind in the first two or three years after I returned to Australia. The glands in my neck would swell every now and again and, each time, I would plummet into the fear of recurrence. Gradually I came to see these occurrences as my reminders. Was I allowing enough time for rest and meditation? Was I nourishing my body, mind and spirit on a daily basis?

Shortly after coming home I established a naturopathic practice. I did this somewhat reluctantly for the experience of living with dying had been a very intense one and the thought of creating a career out of acne, asthma and arthritis held little appeal. However, it was what I was trained to do and I needed to generate an income so that I could create a home for myself and my children, should they wish to live with me again.

Within two weeks of commencing my practice two people with life-threatening illnesses came to see me. Jenny had breast cancer and John had AIDS, and both of them had been told they wouldn't see Christmas; just what I'd been told fifteen months previously. These were people I could understand and relate to. We were fellow travellers walking the same terrain of an uncertain future. We shared our stories, gleaned knowledge and information from one another. We stood together to contemplate our fears and terrors, listened deeply to one another's pain and shared tears of both laughter and despair. Over the ensuing months Jenny and John found peace and the quality of their lives improved. Depression lifted and they both exhibited a greater ability to live one day at a time.

When I heard Jenny's and then John's story I felt deeply alive and able to offer something of value to them. I never set out to work with people with life-threatening illnesses, but over the next few months more and more people began to find their way to my door. After about seven months I was only counselling people with cancer, HIV, AIDS or other life-threatening or life-challenging diseases.

The next ten years I worked from home and often had two hundred or more people through my lounge room each week. They would come for support groups, to learn meditation, for counselling, naturopathic guidance or simply because they were frightened, vulnerable and fragile. My children, who were living with me then, and I fondly referred to our house as the Home for the Bewildered! My work and my life were inextricably entwined.

In 1990 I started a charity called the Quest for Life Foundation so that I could expand the services provided to people with life-threatening illnesses and their loved ones. This enabled me to train more facilitators for support groups and put to good use the volunteers who were keen to offer their services to help others. There is information in the back of this book about the Quest for Life Foundation and how you might support us in our work now.

Through the support groups and my individual counselling we explore and discover all kinds of answers to those fundamental questions about living. Through a willingness to share our stories we begin to find a common path towards healing. Healing is not about finding a cure but about the experience of peace.

So many people have told me my own story over and over again. Their stories contain characters I don't know and the scenes of their lives may differ from my own, but the plot is the same. Each struggles to find peace and a sense of resolution with the past.

In my experience, people who actively participate in their own healing process have an improved quality and, often, quantity of life. As it turned out, Jenny celebrated another two Christmases with her family, and John another five.

We don't need to predict how long another person

will live. I believe that in years to come it will be illegal for a doctor to tell patients at diagnosis how long he or she thinks they have to live. It will be shown that if the person believes the doctor, they will begin to secrete chemicals in their brain that will ensure the doctor's prognosis is correct. These are the chemicals of hopelessness, helplessness and powerlessness. And they are toxic indeed.

People come to me saying their doctor has told them they have a terminal disease. I tell them that terminals are for buses and trains and computers, and that we're people *living* with a life-threatening illness not *dying* with a terminal one. Even if the outcome is the same, what is really important is how we experience that outcome and the life we have to live between now and then.

What stops us from living for now? What gets in the way of us feeling deeply alive and at peace all the time? What do we need to do in order to feel fully alive right now?

Through my contact with people living with life-threatening illnesses I have found that most people seem to face very similar issues even though their backgrounds might be diverse. The diagnosis of a life-threatening illness brings sharply into focus the areas of people's lives that aren't working well or that need attention and resolution. Some of the fundamental questions people can face might be related to how they feel about themselves or those they love, or they might be about purpose and meaning in their lives. Most people aren't afraid of dying but of the process of dying – what's going to happen to me between now and death?

Modern medicine has come a long way in its ability to reduce and often eliminate the physical pain and discomfort that many people with life-threatening illnesses suffer. However, it is wrong to think that physical pain is controllable in everyone; it very much depends on the nature of the pain or the person's ability to deal with their suffering. In addition, many people face emotional, psychological and spiritual pain as they journey with their illness and its consequences.

As a community we hold enormous fear about pain and we want assurances that, should we or someone we love ever be faced with illness, our pain can be eliminated. This perhaps leads to the belief that there should be the option of voluntary euthanasia should a person feel their quality of life is seriously compromised. As a society we accept, indeed encourage, the passive euthanasia of increasing medication to the point where it not only reduces pain but hurries the dying process. However, legalised active voluntary euthanasia where a patient is given a lethal injection which ends their life is a controversial and complex topic.

We have no legislation about who might bring a baby *into* the world nor do we legislate about the necessary interventions to help in the survival of an extremely premature baby. We invest millions of dollars in technology and expertise which ensures the survival of the weakest and yet we withhold the choice for those who are ready and anxious to die as if they're breaking a fundamental law of nature. Modern medicine constantly interferes with nature. As a society we go to endless lengths to stop people from dying, as if to die is the ultimate failure. It is reflected in our language when we say that someone lost the battle with cancer. Yet this is the same society that willingly sends its young people off to fight another nation's war and then celebrates the courage of those who gave their lives for the freedom of others. These contradictions are common and confusing – it's appropriate to die fighting someone else's war but not through individual choice when suffering is intolerable.

For ten years during the early eighties and nineties I facilitated a support and meditation group for hundreds of people with HIV and AIDS at the Albion Street Centre in Sydney. Suicide and euthanasia were discussed almost weekly by group members who were concerned about how their lives might end as their illness took its course. One person with AIDS, George, having attended support groups for many years, chose suicide as a way of completing his life. His relationships were up to date and he had found his peace. George's quality of life had diminished beyond the level most people could tolerate and he consciously chose to end his life with dignity. I don't believe he died defeated by his illness. He chose to die at a time and in a manner that he had considered deeply. Having courageously faced his suffering and eked out whatever growth might have come from his life, he had chosen to die. I could never stand in judgement of someone who made George's choice, and had voluntary euthanasia been available to him, he would most certainly have chosen it.

Voluntary euthanasia has rarely been raised as an option for the many thousands of people with cancer that I have counselled or met through support groups. Perhaps that is because their physical, psychological, emotional and spiritual suffering is openly and freely discussed, explored and understood.

Perhaps here lies a key to our dilemma. I believe that if we are moving towards legislating for voluntary euthanasia we need to improve the emotional, psychological and spiritual comfort and support we give those nearing the end of their life so that it equals the high quality of physical care provided. That is the challenge to our community at this time. Standing beside someone who looks into the dark abyss of suffering with a willingness to feel the pain of our own helplessness to bring relief is a challenge most of us shy away from.

Active voluntary euthanasia is already illegally available to some people in our community. However, we live in an age of open debate and disclosure and we're demanding that what happens behind closed doors becomes embodied in legislation. The complex arguments for and against legalised voluntary euthanasia must continue so that we as a society can clarify how we're going to meet the pain of those who seek an end to their suffering. Most of those in a position to legislate have never looked into the eyes of a person who seeks release from their torment. It is easy to offer an opinion born of the intellect rather than to find compassion and wisdom through venturing into the heart of pain.

How realistic this is considering the society in which we live is yet to be determined. Are we driven by the economics of looking after the sick or by their compassionate care? Is there a balance between the two and who will make the decisions about where that balance lies?

Much of modern medicine is based on what I call the 'fix it, change it, make it better' model, and so it should be. When we have a physical problem we need all the expertise we can get to remedy the situation and restore us to health. This is right and proper and the advances that modern medicine has made in the last century are nothing short of amazing.

However, there's far more to physical healing than just treating the body and its symptoms. The patient's cooperation, willingness to get well, courage, tenacity, hope or other qualities are essential, especially if the treatment or rehabilitation is protracted. As health professionals we can only enter this dimension of healing when we're willing to listen deeply to the person and discover what this illness or trauma means to them.

Much of professional medical training is based upon the belief that practitioners should remain emotionally detached from their patients. This has always seemed a nonsense to me because practitioner and patient are constantly reacting to one another. We all have people we automatically warm to and others we find difficult to like. Also, as a patient myself, I found that the staff who were willing to share something of themselves and their lives were more real and human to me than those whose clinical expertise was undoubted but with whom I felt no rapport. The cleaners, gardeners, handymen and kitchen staff were my particular favourites because they weren't constrained by a code of professional ethics and would chat about the everyday occurrences in their lives.

I believe this lack of real interaction between the health professionals and their patients is a lost opportunity for healing, and that for the health professional it can lead to burnout.

Healing is not just about our physical bodies. There are many who attain a great age but who haven't healed the relationships in their lives or with themselves, and because of this have never found peace. This healing is not dependent on age, health or circumstance, but on a willingness to resolve whatever stands in the way of peace.

People sometimes want something from me that will change their dismal prognosis. They want to know about meditation, visualisation, juices, diet, Kambucha or Essiac tea, crystals, vitamins, psychic surgery, pycnogenol, aloe vera, fasting, intravenous vitamins, chelation and ozone therapies, homeopathy and psychotherapy; anything that might prevent them from dying from their disease.

My focus is always to encourage each person to go all out for peace. When we have peace of mind, we create the very best of environments for healing within our bodies, minds and spirits. If we go all out for a cure and don't achieve it, then we are unlikely to have peace. It is difficult to talk about peace of mind, however, before a person has peace of body. So I use whatever skills and knowledge I have to help a person find peace of body, peace of mind and peace of spirit. This might involve using the physical therapies of diet, vitamins, massage and so on, but it might equally contain the therapy of stories, meditation, forgiveness or visualisation techniques. My focus is not on stopping a person from dying but helping them to live *now*, today. What do they need in order to find peace? For instance, it might be a matter of taking care of their nausea or pain first so that we can then look deeper at some other issue.

When we help people to *really* live then some kind of magic begins to happen and often profound and unexpected changes take place within their bodies.

I believe that our body is our spacesuit for planet earth. We can't have a human experience without a body. We each inhabit our spacesuit, but there comes a time when we return the spacesuit to the elements from which it was formed and move on to other things. It is our responsibility to take good care of the spacesuit during our lifetimes and to see to any repairs or adjustments it might need as we journey along. Sometimes we damage our spacesuit by the way we care for it, perhaps by the inadequate nourishment we've given it, or by our attitudes and beliefs, or by the actions we take or neglect to take.

We need to look at the things that connect us deeply to our inner selves and then make sure those things are happening in our lives. It is no-one else's responsibility to make sure that we find deep peace within ourselves. No-one else is going to come along and fasten your seat belt. It's your responsibility. We can only remind one another about the importance of inner peace and perhaps help each other to find those resources which make that connection possible.

I can't stress strongly enough that it is not simply the seriously ill who need to find a path to peace. We all need to find a way of connecting to the innermost parts of ourselves where we can find resolution and understanding. Many people are forced to find this connection by the threat of illness or the advent of some tragedy or trauma in their lives, but I hope by sharing these stories with you that you can move closer to your own peace, whether you are living with a life-threatening illness or not.

We're constantly teachers and students to one another. If we believe that we're embarked upon a journey of self-discovery and healing, then every encounter with another person is an opportunity to explore and understand who we are and to recognise why we are the way we are. When a person aggravates, irritates or attracts us it can become an opportunity for self-understanding. We can learn so much from each other, if we have the willingness to recognise our responses to situations or people as opportunities to know something about ourselves that we might have otherwise missed. It isn't a matter of whose perception is right or wrong but of how our attitudes, beliefs or judgements have affected our perception and how we can find common ground.

Sometimes, in order to find peace we must venture through the heart of pain. Many people spend their lives running from their feelings because they simply don't know how to address their pain or confusion. We often prefer to fill up our lives with the business of *doing* rather than dealing with the feelings of *being*. It is easier to immerse ourselves in careers, family affairs, commitments and responsibilities than to look within ourselves and find resolution to our fears, self-doubts, grief or whatever stands in the way of peace. But we are, after all, human beings rather than human doings, and if peace is to be our goal then we must each address ourselves to its blossoming in our lives. As peace blossoms within us our lives become transformed and we bring a new sense of joy and love to every aspect of our being. Then we can live without the clutter of the past undermining the peace that is possible in each present moment.

The people in the following stories have been my teachers, my friends, my mentors. They have helped me to heal myself of the prejudices and judgements which block my own path to peace. For many years, I railed at the black hole within myself believing it had the potential to destroy me. They have helped me to discover it as the wellspring of my creativity, inspiration and intuition, and for that I am forever in their debt.

KATE

It has been said by people older and wiser than I am that if we take the time to listen, children are among our best teachers. They have the ability to go straight to the heart of a matter – no frills, no pretensions and no saying what they think we want to hear. Children have impacted very deeply on my life and I am grateful to have met some of these teachers so early in my career as a counsellor.

Kate was ten years old and had cancer of the heart muscle. She had come to me for counselling as her prognosis was poor. Kate radiated life and love. She always lit up the room when she walked in with her mother, Julie. Kate had a remarkable spirit and took the limitations of her illness in her stride. She would say things like: 'I'm sad that I can't go to school any more. I suppose Jesus will teach me everything I need to know when I get to heaven.' Kate was blessed with a particularly close and loving family. She drew strength from them and they encouraged and supported her in her faith that she was loved deeply by God.

Kate had to travel many miles to visit me and one particular day she brought a picture she had drawn. The picture depicted the cartoon character Garfield with three coloured hearts inside the bubble of his thoughts. She told me she had actually drawn two pictures but when she put them on her windowsill the wind had blown the other one away. She said she would draw me an identical one and send it to me. I asked her what was in the other picture. She replied that it was exactly the same but that the hearts were all shattered down the middle.

Being a counsellor I said to her that perhaps the wind was telling her she had no need of broken hearts. She shook her head and replied: 'No, Petrea, you don't understand. Sometimes hearts have got to break before they heal.'

Kate's second picture duly arrived. For years I've had the two Garfields pinned to the cork board in my counselling room.

In the first years of counselling people with life-threatening illnesses I was afraid that my own heart would break. I was constantly confronted with stories of pain, loss and heartache. I would often sit in my office at the end of a long, long day and reflect upon the stories I had heard. My heart would be heavy as I'd think: 'Why does it have to hurt so much to be human? Why do parents have to lose their children? What is the purpose of suffering?' I struggled to find any sense or meaning in the pain of the stories I listened to all day long, day after day.

Eventually, I experienced massive burnout. A friend with leukaemia gave me the keys to her holiday apartment in Queensland and insisted that I take a break. On my arrival I had turned on the television just as a program on the gaol system in Australia began. They were talking about prisoners with AIDS and I thought, 'Who is going to look after them?' and I began to weep uncontrollably. I continued crying for the next ten days except for when the sleep of emotional exhaustion overtook me. I grappled more and more deeply with the questions of human suffering. I had an intellectual knowledge gleaned from my religious and other studies, but the raw emotion of my daily exposure to human suffering was overwhelming. I questioned my motives for working with these people and their families. Why do I need to be needed? Why is there so much pain in the world? What is it that I want to offer these people? What is it they want from me?

Out of my questioning came the realisation that I often saw my clients as dying people and had given them an unhealthy importance in my life. I realised that this had come about because of 'survivor guilt'. I was meant to have died and my remission gave me an unsettling sense of living on borrowed time. Early on in my counselling, when I was relatively unknown for my work, my diary was fully booked six weeks ahead. I constantly had phone calls from people who were given less than that time to live, so I squeezed them in on Saturday or Sunday. I was counselling people six days a week and visiting them, if they were too sick to get to me, in their homes, hospitals or hospices on Sundays. I had again made other people's needs more important than my own.

People say you feel better for a good cry. I didn't feel one jot better knowing that I was returning to the same amount of pain and suffering. On my drive home from Queensland I thought about what I needed to do in order not only to survive my work, but also to thrive and grow from it. I realised that I needed to listen to myself as keenly as I endeavoured to listen to my clients. Some simple strategies that have served me well came out of this revelation. I found and put in place the things I knew would deeply nurture and nourish me. These included my daily early morning walks along the beach and finding someone who could provide professional supervision in my work. I needed the same safe space for myself that I tried to create for my clients. I found a wonderful psychiatrist who I saw weekly for the next eight or nine years. I refined my diet a little to include daily fruit or vegetable juices, and I made more time for music, nature and solitude. By the time I arrived home I knew the ingredients I needed to create a more balanced life for myself. I had held many people in my arms as they had died. At what point did they stop living and start dying? I no longer saw my clients as dying people but people very much alive and living. This changed perception proved to be a major key in the way in which I was able to work from then on.

On my return, Kate's pictures and her wise words took on a new and deeper meaning.

In ten short years Kate had gleaned what was truly important in life. She knew that we sometimes have to venture through the heart of what is painful in order to find a deep and unshakeable peace.

The inability to deal with serious illness and the death of a child can often cause a marriage to break down. This whole situation can be exacerbated by simple geographic difficulties. If a family lives a long way from a major children's hospital, there are the added strains of a split family as one parent accompanies the child to hospital for treatments and the other parent continues with their work and perhaps the additional care of other children. This separation means added expense, lack of emotional closeness, and the absence of the very person a parent most needs by his or her side. Illness and death put tremendous strains on family relationships and sadly sixty-five per cent of marriages break down after the death of a child.

Kate's family negotiated all these difficulties with determination and great faith. The warmth and love in their home was the foundation upon which they dealt with the pain and suffering of Kate's illness and death.

Not long before she died Kate reached out to take her parents' hands and said: 'I want you to love each other the way you've loved me.'

I believe that it was the depth of love and faith within her family that enabled Kate to learn such valuable and profound lessons about what is truly important in life.

Kate's life continues to be an inspiration to me and to the many who have heard her story. Kate learnt and then taught others that love heals all; that we are precious to one another, and that out of suffering can come wisdom, a greater capacity to love and a deep certainty about life built on faith and hope.

When I had finished writing Kate's story for this book I faxed through a copy for her parents, Ray and Julie, to read. The following was their reply.

> *We were all moved by what you wrote and a flood of memories came back as we sat together reading in the lounge. Actually, at the exact moment Ray was reading the fax, brilliant rays of coloured sunshine shone in on his face. They were coming in through a crystal pelican that was Kates and which we have in our sunroom – a little comforting sign and one of her approval, we feel. I am sure nothing happens in this life by chance and it is truly a wonderful journey to travel with all sorts of experiences along the way. Out of our experience we have grown and matured so much and have come to a stage where we are extremely happy and positive people.*

DON

One of the many ways I have been inspired in my work has been through the courage and selflessness I have seen in people helping one another. No matter how desperate their situation, the desire to understand and support has been paramount in these often angry, hurt and bewildered people who have healed through their dedication to others.

To many, to heal means to cure. To me, healing is about finding deep and unshakeable peace. No matter how long or short the life, to go in peace is surely the goal, and if one can assist others to experience that same peace, it is heroism indeed.

Some years ago, through the Quest for Life Foundation, I ran a very busy support centre from my home in Sydney. We had a core staff of three people and relied upon volunteers to help provide many of our services. In addition to the support groups and counselling, we would also receive hundreds of phone calls from distressed people who were newly diagnosed or dealing with the difficulties of their or their loved one's illness. Many of our callers were frightened, depressed, angry or despairing, and they needed a special kind of person to help them through their anguish.

Don was one of our most loved and valued volunteers. For many years he was a participant in our support and meditation groups as he had AIDS. In addition, each week he would come to our centre and answer the telephone. Don calmly and compassionately listened to every caller's troubles. Unbeknown to them, he was himself terribly affected by AIDS and was plagued with unrelenting diarrhoea which left him both debilitated and painfully thin. Yet his ability to love and be available to others was extraordinary.

There finally came a time when Don was no longer able to venture outside the tiny apartment he shared with his partner. They lived up a long and steep flight of stairs which he could no longer manage and the problems with his body made it essential to remain close to the bathroom. Many would say his quality of life was abysmal and yet I never heard Don complain.

I used to visit him whenever I could as his company was always pleasant and his contacts with the outside world were few. On one occasion we were sitting in his lounge talking about how he felt about his weakness and his impending death. Don had a deep serenity which we all drew strength from, and he told me: 'Sometimes, when I sit here, the smell of freshly-brewed coffee wafts up through the window from the cafe downstairs. Sometimes I hear snatches of conversation from the street below. Occasionally two little sparrows sit on the garage roof outside my window and sing to one another. I can't imagine heaven can be any nicer than where I am right now.'

We can rail at the world and lament the things we cannot do. Don could have focused on the fact that he could no longer leave the house to attend the theatre, the opera or social events. He could have made himself miserable by bemoaning his many losses. Instead, Don chose to rejoice in what gave him pleasure and in this way he found his peace. It is a challenge indeed to see our glass as half full when our suffering is so great.

JOSH

There is increasing discussion about death and dying in our community. Not so many years ago, death was a taboo subject, and talk of funerals, coffins, wills, cremation or burial was considered morbid. Nowadays there are lectures, workshops, books and tapes about death readily available to everyone. The information and knowledge that we've gleaned from other religious traditions – such as those described in *The Tibetan Book of Living and Dying* by Sogyal Rinpoche for example – have led to new perceptions about dying well.

Unfortunately, armed with this knowledge, many people then make judgements about whether a person has had a 'good' death. This can certainly include health professionals who, by and large, want their patients to die with peace and serenity, having resolved whatever they might need to in their lives. Not all deaths fit this stereotype, and I believe we must be very careful about leaping to the conclusion that someone has somehow not measured up to our preconceived ideas of what dying well means.

One of my very first clients was a young man with leukaemia. The first time Josh came to see me, he struggled with the telling of his story. He was painfully shy and seemed completely at a loss as to how to cope with his illness and the debility he experienced as a result of his treatments. Though he would cooperate with the hospital by turning up to his appointments, he wouldn't speak to the social worker who tried to give him support and encouragement. When he returned to his bedsitter after each treatment, he would climb into bed and sleep for days at a time, taking little care of himself. In view of the fact that he wasn't eating well, the social worker despaired of his ability to withstand the aggressiveness of his treatments. She knew that Josh had a deep suspicion of the medical establishment so she suggested that, in addition to his treatments, he come to me for naturopathic counselling.

Initially we talked about some easy ways for him to nourish himself on the days when he didn't feel up to eating. But I was keen to penetrate his shyness and lethargy to see what his deeper issues might be.

Each session I had with him felt like drawing teeth. He found it enormously difficult to articulate his feelings as they seemed to run so deep. I asked him if he could illustrate for me the difficulty he seemed to have in expressing how he felt. Josh described it to me by comparing it with the doctors trying to extract his bone marrow. Some of his marrow had solidified, becoming nothing more than scar tissue, whilst what else remained was sludgy and difficult to remove. A more apt description hardly seemed possible and I had the distinct impression that Josh's will to live lay deeply covered by emotional scarring.

In one session Josh told me he came from a deeply conservative Jewish background and that his attempts to resist his mother's constant badgering were futile. She wanted him to succeed in life and she constantly gave him advice about every decision he had to make. She disapproved of his choices in women and felt that none of them were suitable for him.

Though he had moved interstate to remove himself from her physically, he felt that she had inculcated her judgements and beliefs into his very being. He felt there was no escape from her; yet much of what she believed, he too found strengthening. As is often the case within families, an undermining of one's sense of self can be transmitted through the subtlety of our interaction; so that it isn't so much what a person says but the way in which they say it through their body language, behaviour, choice of words, inflection, emphasis, hesitation or what is left unsaid that becomes important.

When Josh was diagnosed with leukaemia it took every ounce of his being to resist his mother's desire to move in and care for him. He minimised both his diagnosis and prognosis and glossed over how terrible he felt. He told me he'd rather die than have her look after him. Besides, there simply wasn't any space for her in his bedsitter and the thought of her there crowded out any possibility of his own independent existence.

At the same time as I was seeing Josh, I was also counselling a young woman who could not have been more different to him. Lynne had a brain tumour in her pituitary gland. Although it was a benign tumour, it was still life threatening for if it continued to grow, it would interfere with the gland's proper functioning. She was on medication to control its growth and her dream was to reduce the medication so that she could have a baby. Her doctors had told her without any compromise that if she were ever to have a child, the hormones produced in pregnancy would reactivate the tumour and change her prognosis dramatically.

Lynne was a free-spirited young woman who believed that all the things she was doing in addition to her medical treatment allowed the real possibility of her being able to fulfil her dream of motherhood. These things involved diet, juices, meditation and visualisation. Most of the time she was very cheery, though there were times when she would express her fears about not being able to have a child and frustration at the other limitations the tumour placed upon her.

Lynne never hesitated to express how she felt or what she thought and I believed it would be beneficial for both her and Josh if they were to meet. I sometimes felt at a loss to help Josh extricate himself from the lifelong patterns that bound him. I must confess that I thought he would be the main recipient of anything positive to come out of their contact – a belief I discovered to be quite erroneous as I witnessed their deepening friendship.

Lynne and Josh were the sole members of our very first support group. At that time support groups were virtually nonexistent in Australia and there were no guidelines by which to run them. Over the first few weeks the three of us fashioned our own guidelines for the effective running of a cancer support group. We decided upon four points to be followed for the smooth running of the group and these are the very same guidelines that we have continued to use in each of our support groups since.

1. Confidentiality. This means that we don't speak outside of the group about anyone who attends the group nor about anything that is discussed.
2. We listen one hundred per cent when someone is talking. That means one person talking at a time, but it also means *really* hearing the other person's story rather than our *reaction* to what they're saying.
3. We don't judge each other. If someone feels miserable, depressed, suicidal, peaceful, positive or negative, we don't tell them that they shouldn't feel like that. If *that's* how you feel, then *that's* how you feel, and telling someone they shouldn't feel that way is less than no help.
4. We stay with how we feel rather than what we think. For many of us this is difficult because we are so used to living up to everyone else's or our own standards that sometimes it's really hard to know how we actually *feel*.

Once satisfied with how the group should be run and its function, we plunged into the enlightening experience of sharing our stories in an environment made safe by our guidelines.

During the first few months, more and more people wanted to attend and before long I was facilitating two groups during the day and one group at night.

Lynne gained as much from her contact with Josh as he did from her. She became a little more thoughtful and less cavalier, and Josh's humour resurfaced in a distinctly black way that we all enjoyed. Only those who live at life's edge can enjoy the fullness of black humour and Josh became a master of the unpalatable, the tacky, the bizarre and the unspeakable. He would listen intently to whatever was being said and, at a time always appropriate, would drop in a remark that dissolved any tension and reduced us to tears of laughter. During a two-hour group we'd lurch from one emotion to another and yet, by the group's end, we'd feel enlivened, encouraged and fortified enough by one another to continue with our individual journeys.

After about three months of attending each weekly group, Josh sheepishly told us that he had fallen in love for the first time. We were delighted for him and chided him about being a dark horse and keeping this new friendship from us. He grinned shyly, but there was a definite twinkle in his eye which I hadn't seen before. He was keen for Lauren to attend the group with him and we looked forward to meeting her. However, as the weeks progressed, Lauren didn't come to the group and each week Josh conveyed to us her excuse for her absence.

Initially his health improved. His new-found love had coincided with his leukaemia going into remission. We laughed with him about how sex as therapy could make your cells sing. Lynne wondered out loud whether it might make his bone marrow juicier and less stodgy. We all giggled at the image.

Though Josh was clearly disappointed that Lauren could not get to the group, he always accepted her excuses and never put pressure on her to attend. This was very different from Lynne's forthright approach and she asked Josh why he didn't tell Lauren how important it was for him that she should come. Josh was unused to expressing his needs even in this new relationship, but he resolved to explain to Lauren that he needed her to come to the group so she could understand more fully what he was experiencing.

The following week Josh told us that they had had their first argument. Lauren didn't want to come to the group and made the excuse that he could speak more freely if she wasn't present. Josh felt deeply hurt by this. He told us that the group had become his lifeline and for the first time in his memory he was beginning to form his own opinions and beliefs. This was a healing beyond even his expectations and we were deeply touched to be part of his journey.

Lauren had enjoyed looking after Josh when he had been frail and needed support; however, as he became stronger and more independent she began to find faults with the way he was conducting his recovery.

One night, quite late, Josh rang me extremely distraught. He and Lauren had had an almighty row and she had stormed off into the night. I asked him what they had fought over and he told me that Lauren thought he wasn't trying hard enough to maintain his remission.

I was loathe to see Josh disappear once more within himself and, after talking for a little while, he agreed to come and see me early the next morning.

Josh turned up for his appointment looking a little dishevelled and obviously in need of more sleep. He talked about the early days of their romance when Lauren had been so attentive and caring towards him. They had shared stories and laughter and she seemed to understand that much of him was deeply wounded by his upbringing. She treated these tender parts of him with love and respect.

As he had regained his health and independence Lauren had taken it upon herself to find out about more and more alternative therapies which might benefit him. She insisted that he drink the juices she made for him and that when she was at work he make them for himself. She had become more and more particular about what and when he ate and had enrolled them both in a course on astrology, a subject they both enjoyed but which he had no desire to study. He felt his life was once more being taken over by someone who thought they knew what was best for him.

It quickly became apparent to us both that Josh had fallen for someone very much like his mother. To start with this hadn't been readily obvious and Josh had enjoyed the fun and laughter and the care Lauren had taken of him; but now he felt that she could only cope with him when he was in need of her and that this was an unbalanced way to have a relationship. He wasn't sure that he had the courage to withstand her strong beliefs but resolved to try to talk to her.

The following day Josh haemorrhaged internally and was rushed to hospital. For the first time, by his bedside, Lauren met Josh's mother. Lauren was wary of her because of the many stories Josh had told her, and Josh's mother was clearly distinctly unimpressed with her son's choice of partner.

Josh did not regain consciousness. As the morning of the second day dawned, his mother and Lauren seemed only to antagonise each other further. Each one appeared to want to outdo the other in the way in which she cared for Josh. The stress and worry over him and their lack of sleep didn't help what was fast becoming a fairly volatile situation. Josh's mother talked loudly in his ear, telling him to relax. Lauren told her in an irritated manner, 'Josh isn't deaf, and don't you know that hearing is the last faculty to go?' And then, 'Josh *is* relaxed, and what would you know about helping him to relax anyway?' The two women tried to contain their dislike of each other but it deteriorated into an ugly argument in which accusations were hurled.

Suddenly Josh began to yell, though there was no physical reason for him to do so. It was unlikely that he was in pain or that his shouting had anything to do with his physical deterioration, but his yelling drowned out the argument between the women and made it a nonsense. He screamed and yelled and then continued with loud groans which made any conversation between his mother and his girlfriend impossible. Josh kept it up until he died half an hour later.

The staff on the ward and Josh's mother and girlfriend were devastated by the manner in which Josh left but I wonder. We can presume to know too much if we quickly decide that a death like Josh's was a disaster.

Perhaps Josh found his voice for the first time and spoke from the depths of his being about who he was and what he felt in a language more articulate than mere words. Perhaps. I am too wary of making a judgement about another's experience to say definitely, but I like to think that my summation contains an element of truth.

We are often quick to label or pigeonhole people or their experiences. Perhaps we would all benefit by being more content to live with the mystery of the questions. Many people seek answers as a way of convincing themselves that they have control over life or that they possess an understanding of why life unfolds in the way it does.

The group mourned Josh and was taken aback by the suddenness of his deterioration and death. Lynne in particular struggled to come to terms with the manner in which Josh died, but she drew comfort and reassurance from the idea that I voiced to her. Lynne felt intuitively that it was right and gradually we came to talk of him more easily and remembered his humour and the support his presence always gave us.

To this day the hardest part of my job is to tell a support group that one of its members has died. It's awful to be the bearer of such sad tidings. I know the information is going to confront people with not only the sadness of the loss of someone they loved, but also with the fragility of their own life and the possible outcome of their own disease.

Over the years we have developed a ritual which enables us to deal effectively with the grief we all experience when a much-loved member of the support group dies.

After talking to the group and giving them whatever information I might have about the person's death, we discuss for a while any thoughts or feelings we might have. In talking things through we remember what it was that we loved in the person, and we struggle with the incomprehensibility of the fact that this person was in the group only last week or last month and how sudden their death seems to us.

When we have finished talking we join hands, close our eyes lightly and bring all of our awareness into the present moment by connecting it to our physical senses. Being aware of our weight and posture, the pressure of the chair, the floor, the air and our clothing against the skin, and all the sounds inside and outside the room helps us to connect with the present moment.

The mind is always projecting into the future or chewing over the past; seldom is it fully alive and aware in the present moment. The body is always in the present, and for this reason it is precious. It serves as an anchor to bring us back to what *is* and away from our mind which flies in so many directions.

Once everyone is focused in this way I ask them to imagine that the members of the group form the base of a rainbow, as if all the rainbow's iridescent colours surround and envelop each one. I'll explain this a little further in Jenny's story. We then take a moment to breathe in our favourite colours; then we imagine the person who has died in the centre of the rainbow, as if they stand before us.

We reflect upon the qualities that endeared them to us. Perhaps their sense of humour, their tenacity, their courage or love, or whatever it might be that was precious in them. We take a moment to each say silently in our minds whatever might be in our hearts that we wish to convey to that person. Then we listen to what they might say to us in reply. We extend a rainbow from our hearts to the heart of the person who has died, and we allow the qualities that we valued to flow back over that rainbow bridge as their gifts to us. We extend our love and blessings to them to carry them on their way, then we imagine them dissolving into light.

This ritual gives us a tangible way in which to grieve and express ourselves, and it has brought a lot of comfort to us all over the years.

Two years after Josh's death, Lynne fell in love and she and her partner Paul decided to bring their first child into the world. Her doctors still spoke darkly of the consequences of her decision, but she held fast to her long-held desire and the following year her son was born. One of the names they gave their firstborn was Joshua.

EMMA

Sometimes it is easier to communicate through a symbolic language than through words. This can be especially so for children who haven't yet learnt the words to articulate their fears and concerns. However, this symbolic language is not confined to children: many of us find it easier to express ourselves through symbols rather than words, though it is not always easy to read this symbolic language and we often need help in deciphering it.

A Tuesday afternoon brought seven-year-old Emma and her mother to my rooms. Emma's oncologist had recommended me because Emma was suffering anticipatory nausea for several days before she had chemotherapy. This is not at all uncommon in both children and adults who've been having chemotherapy for some time. Even the thought of going to the hospital made Emma's tummy churn.

Emma had a cancer in the bone in her lower leg which was going to necessitate her having her left leg amputated at the knee on Friday of that same week. So it was hardly surprising the thought of hospital made her feel sick.

She was small for her age and was reluctant to have yet another health professional involved in her care. We talked about the foods which would be helpful to eat and the ones which might make her feel yucky. She showed little interest.

I tried to turn it into a bit of a game and told her to imagine she had little people in her tummy and that when she ate greasy, overrefined foods or drinks these little people would put up their umbrellas and wait, very unhappily, for it all to pass. Emma gave me a withering look, 'Give me a break' written all over her pale little face. Undaunted, I continued with my story, telling her that when she sent down fruit and vegies, fish and chicken, and so on, they just about had a party in her tummy because these were the foods they needed and wanted to make her well.

Finally, with an air of having to describe the most elementary of facts to a slow learner, Emma said, 'I know I've got people in my body.' Her mother and I contained our surprise as she continued. 'They're the ones who do all the work and make me move. I've got them in my arms and legs and everywhere.'

Suddenly this child who had been so quiet became animated as she described the intricate workings of her body. Without drawing breath she told us, 'In my head there's a man who sits on a high stool and behind him there's a screen and he projects onto the screen what he wants to have happen in my body and in front of him there's a big semicircular table with people with phones and they look at the screen and see what's meant to happen in my body and then they ring up the part of my body and tell it to do it.' She finally drew breath only to continue: 'There are little people with pulleys who make it all happen. Look, you watch.' She lifted her arm, concentrated for a moment and then bent it at the elbow. 'See, they're doing it.'

I agreed that this was truly amazing as she went through various parts of her body and showed me how the little people made her eyes blink, her legs move and so on.

I found it curious that Emma spoke of a man in her head until one day, years later, I saw in a children's book the picture she had described in detail.

After a time, I asked her, 'What does the man in your head think about what's happening in your left leg?'

Emma's eyes immediately overflowed with tears and she blurted out, 'He thinks he's done something wrong because he can't get through on the telephone!'

'He thinks it's his fault?' I asked. She nodded emphatically.

I continued, 'Emma the cancer in your leg has nothing to do with him. It's not his fault. These are just a bad batch of cells and you have to let the doctors take them away.'

Suddenly she heaved a huge sigh, closed her eyes and said, 'He says to say you're a friend.'

We talked a little more about the necessity of surgery

and then I asked her whether the man in her head might be able to get through on the telephone with messages of thanks to her left leg. Thanks for being there for the past seven years because she had learnt how to walk and run, and she chimed in with, 'And how to swim and ski.' Once more she closed her eyes and became quiet. 'Yes!' she said after a moment, 'He says I can.'

I asked Emma to ask him whether she could get through with another message. Could he let them know that there was about to be a big change at the knee and that all the wires would be cut? Soon she would have another leg which wouldn't be anything like her present one but it would work really well when she got used to it.

Again she closed her eyes and confirmed that yes, she could get through with that message also.

Finally it was decided that for the next three nights before her surgery she would send messages of love and thanks to her leg as she prepared her knee for the coming changes.

At the end of our session I said to Emma, 'So how are you feeling about the surgery now?'

She replied thoughtfully: 'I'm kind of sad and I'm kind of happy. I'm sad because I'm going to lose an old friend, but I'm happy because I know when *it* goes, I can live.'

In her own way and given a language in which she could articulate her concerns and apprehensions, Emma stumbled upon peace and resolution.

I have a number of magic wands in my office. You may have seen smaller versions of them. These are sealed tubes filled with stars, moons and glitter in coloured oils which move slowly up and down inside the cylinder. The two I have are just under a metre long. When a child is to have a bone-marrow transplant or an amputation, I let them borrow one of my 'grandmother' wands to take into hospital with them. I tell them that all the love and healing from all the smaller wands around the world go back to the grandmother wands at night, and that if they hold onto the wand and close their eyes, they can imagine all that love and healing flowing into their bodies.

Emma happily took the grandmother wand with her when she left at the end of our time together. I visited her early on Friday morning before she was due to have her surgery. I found her lying in her hospital bed with her eyes closed, a serene look on her face, holding onto the grandmother wand which was almost the same size as she was.

Several years have passed and Emma continues to thrive. She is at present training for the 2000 Winter Olympics.

COLIN

When a person makes an appointment to see me for the first time, I am usually unaware of their physical condition. A pencilled name and sometimes a diagnosis in a diary gives no indication of who this person might be, nor how long ago their diagnosis was made. Sometimes a person comes to see me who really should not be out of bed. It can show the degree of desperation they feel if someone so ill travels such an uncomfortable journey to my door.

One such young man was Colin. I was very distressed to find him and his distraught wife in my waiting room. Colin was dreadfully thin, weak, deathly pale and sweating with intense pain. We half carried him into my office and made him as comfortable as possible, propping him on cushions and elevating his swollen feet on a footstool. His extremities were icy cold even though the summer breeze that blew softly in from the window was balmy, warm and fragrant from the jasmine growing outside. Colin could barely speak because of his agony, so his young wife, Julie, told me their story.

She and Colin had met at their local church and had been together for three happy years. They had never had an argument until recently when Colin had become more and more withdrawn and irritable. They had been married just over a year and Julie was pregnant with their first child. Six months ago Colin had been diagnosed with bowel cancer but had not seen a doctor since and had undergone no treatment. His diagnosis had been confirmed by a biopsy after he had complained of bleeding from the bowel. I contained both my surprise and my anguish at his condition and gently enquired why they had made the choices they had about his treatment.

Their story was not unusual, though it certainly was extreme. Many people fall into the trap of trying to earn their recovery, believing that if they can only find the right combination of therapies then they will be able to undo the cause of their disease. This thinking is quite popular in our society at present and the worst misunderstanding of this philosophy is that we create our illnesses in order to learn some spiritual lesson from them. Hence, if we follow this thinking, if we can really learn the lesson, then we won't die.

This thinking is far more common than one might expect. It is not far removed from the vengeful God of the Old Testament who visits afflictions upon those who have erred in their behaviour or thinking. Certainly in the early days of the epidemic many people smugly believed that AIDS was the punishment inflicted by a homophobic god. Likewise, many people believe that their cancer is directly caused by some difficulty they have had in their lives or that they are responsible for its creation because of their beliefs or attitudes.

This is a complex area and is often grossly oversimplified by the proponents of this philosophy. It can serve as a terrible judgement and certainly doesn't facilitate the experience of deeply joining together in our humanity. There is often a hidden agenda which says, 'If you eat the right foods, forgive the past, meditate for hours a day, drink your vegetable juices, take your vitamins and only focus on the "positive", then you might not die of your disease.' Those who believe this thinking and who are healthy might use this philosophy as a way of reassuring themselves that the terrible illness that has happened to someone else certainly won't happen to them. Or, if it did, that *they'd* know the way to recovery.

Julie and Colin attended a church that was very much grounded in the belief that illness is a sign of the devil at work and that in order to be healed, one must vanquish the devil through prayer and fasting. To choose surgery, treatment or pain relief was no more than pandering to the devil and would not be tolerated. If a person's faith was strong enough, the devil would be eliminated and health would be restored. If the person died, it was clearly because of a lack of faith in the power of God.

My heart broke for these two young people who clearly loved one another very much and were trying to live according to their beliefs. I wondered if they realised just how close Colin was to dying. He spoke a little of the anguish he felt in letting down Julie and their unborn child because his faith was insufficient to carry him through. He said that he felt a failure because his declining health and his unrelenting pain were grim reminders of his lack of faith.

I felt tearful myself with the terrible pain – physical, emotional and spiritual – that their belief system had caused. How could I proceed to undo some of these cherished beliefs in a way they might accept, and was it my place to do so? I shared with them some of my own journey and chose stories that I felt would have some meaning for them. One of them concerned the 'spiritual healing' I received a couple of months after my diagnosis.

My mother was a keen member of our local Anglican church and asked me whether I would consider having a laying on of hands by the parish priest. I had grown away from orthodox religion some years previously, having found a much deeper satisfaction in meditation and eastern philosophies. However, I was keenly aware that this ritual would bring comfort to my mother and I half-heartedly agreed to participate.

I met with the pastor, John Seddon, of Saint Luke's church in Mosman and was deeply touched by his compassion and faith in the power of God's love to bring about healing. We discussed my spiritual beliefs at that time and how they differed from the dogma of the mainstream church. I didn't believe that Christ had died for my sins but that he showed the way in which we might each find the power of love and forgiveness within ourselves and thus transform our lives. At the end of our meeting John agreed that I might benefit from the laying on of hands. The service was to be held the following Sunday after evensong and I dutifully appeared, though my mother's and John's faith far outweighed my own.

As I approached the altar at the conclusion of evensong I offered up a prayer asking that whatever blessings might be forthcoming from this ritual be directed to my mother whose anguish about my brother's suicide had only been compounded by my illness and possible death. When I knelt at the communion rail I found myself beside two elderly gentlemen who were there, like me, for healing. Something in the simplicity of their faith moved me and I felt an extraordinary outflowing of love and compassion to these two men I'd never met.

When John anointed my forehead and palms with the sign of the cross I was immobilised by a powerful radiance that I can only describe as pure love. I immediately tried to retreat from its presence, believing that I was unworthy to receive it. I felt my heart was too full of darkness to allow such a light into it. It was as if love perceived my quandary and stood firm. This tussle continued in my mind for what seemed a long time.

Finally I realised that the only thing that ever stops us from experiencing love is what we hold in our minds – our beliefs, judgements, desires and perceptions. To let go of guilt and shame and to forgive oneself can seem an insurmountable challenge. I was the cause of my own distress. There was no-one to blame, no-one had caused my beliefs. They were the sum total of my reactions to life's experiences.

If we can be willing to let go of everything that stands in the way of love, then peace and love can become our reality. It was as simple as that. Simple is not always easy though! This experience became one of the guiding lights in my journey towards peace and healing. I realised that I didn't need to earn my recovery, that whether I lived or died, what really mattered was a simple surrender into peace and love.

Colin and Julie listened intently to my story and seemed to gain something from it. We talked about how we sometimes use our body and its health as a marker of how well we might be going with our attempts at healing. We spoke about healing and whether it was possible to find healing and yet not remain in a body. Colin could see that his beliefs were separating him from the experience of peace and that his irritation with Julie and his body only compounded his sense of failure as a loving person. I asked Colin what would be the easiest thing for him to do right now. He answered that to be free of pain and to let go would be 'heaven'.

It is a paradox that we sometimes choose to live in hell believing it is the path to heaven.

As I continued to share stories with them, the atmosphere in the room became lighter and we were able to perceive together a more compassionate and loving way of spirituality. One which left aside guilt and embraced forgiveness as a path to peace. Most of us will agree that forgiveness brings peace; yet do we forgive effortlessly? I pointed out that the Old Testament is focused on justice, vengeance and retribution because it is focused on the survival of the tribe. The New Testament, on the other hand, speaks of a higher path to peace through compassion, love, wisdom, mercy and forgiveness as we make an individual journey towards wholeness.

During our time together, Colin had reached for Julie's hand and she had shifted her chair so that they were as close together as physically possible. It seemed that a huge weight had lifted from both of them and that their separate struggles were at an end. They were one again. Though Colin was very exhausted, he told Julie that there were many things he wanted to share with her.

Colin and Julie had travelled more than two hours across Sydney to see me and I was loathe to see them on their way without some adequate pain relief for Colin.

I called a friend who's a GP and she came immediately. Colin gratefully accepted the morphine she offered and, once he was more comfortable, he and Julie embarked upon their journey home.

Julie called me early the next morning to tell me that Colin had died peacefully at 2 a.m. When they had arrived home they had both lain down upon their bed. With his physical, emotional and spiritual pain released, Colin had curled up in her arms and talked of his love for her and their soon to be born son. He reassured her that he would watch over them both and that, until they met again, his love would surround her. Julie stroked his head with great tenderness and told him to journey well. She reassured him that their child would know his father by the stories she would tell of him.

BELLA

Many people approach illness with the feeling that they have to earn their recovery. They have an underlying belief that if they do all the right things – meditate, never miss a juice, take vitamins and herbs, and so on – then maybe they will pass the test and their reward will be that they get well. This bargaining attitude stems from fear. The old fear of not being good enough. The fear of some perceived standard which many people feel they have to meet, yet don't think they have what it takes to do so.

When we are willing to change, to embrace what is new and unexplored, life can become an adventure. To continue with the old criterion of 'Do I have what it takes?' is to perpetuate a pattern all too familiar to some of us. A lot of people are high achievers and may well fall into the trap of finding a diet or other program so rigorous that it almost makes failure a certainty.

Bella, who was confined to a wheelchair, had flown across the country by private jet to consult with me. She arrived with her husband who appeared to be very attentive to her needs. He declined to join us for her consultation in the belief that she wanted to have this time alone with me.

Bella had had cancer for three and a half years and her doctors had recently told her that she only had weeks to live. She felt utterly desperate as she had travelled the world in search of a cure. For three-quarters of an hour she spoke of her medical history and the many orthodox and alternative treatments she had pursued both within Australia and overseas. As she spoke I listened attentively but with rising panic because she knew far more than I about alternative treatments. I looked serene and peaceful on the outside but I was thinking, 'What can I tell her that she doesn't already know?' and 'It'll have to be something good because she has come all this way to see me.' I knew she was desperate and she had told me I was her last hope.

However, I believe that if a person is in my office then that's precisely where they're meant to be. Panicking about what I might say to Bella only stopped me from being present with her. Worrying about my response was keeping my focus on me and leaving her unheard in any deep sense. People give out all kinds of information about themselves but we need to be intensely present with them in order to hear, feel, smell and see the messages that they offer to us. With these often unspoken messages we can glean far more about a person than seems readily apparent.

Our bodies are always in the present. They are never in the future, nor in the past, and, as I have already said, one of the most effective ways of connecting deeply with the present moment is to focus all our attention on the senses. It is impossible to panic and be completely present at the same time. When we are deeply connected to the present moment our intuition can begin to function well and that still small voice can be heard. I have often been surprised by the depth and clarity of the insights that have come as a result of this simple practice. It's as if we have the ability to tune into a deeper level of communication.

I brought myself wholeheartedly back into the present and focused my absolute attention on Bella and the story she was telling me. Her entire day was governed by the clock. She was taking more juices, vitamins and other pills than you could find in a health food shop and her diet was entirely made up of raw foods.

'I'm sick to *death* of the diet and all the pills,' Bella said, 'but I know they're my only hope.'

We talked about the foods she missed and they all seemed quite innocuous. This lady had *doing* down to a fine art, but had not ventured much into the land of *being*. Her whole day was governed by her 'healing program' and yet she had no peace. She was meditating with one of my tapes three times every day, and enjoying it, but that too was done for a prescribed length of time and with a sense of duty rather than simply for the pleasure of it.

The 'prescription' I gave her that day might sound quite ludicrous to most people. I suggested three things to her which not only surprised her but astounded me.

I told her that she could throw away her clock and her vitamins and herbs and all the books she'd ever read about cancer. I suggested she eat whatever she liked and to forget about her juices unless she felt like one. The key was to consume only the things she *felt* like eating rather than the things she thought she *should* be eating. Bella looked a bit dubious about the dietary suggestions but when I continued with the next idea she crumpled in her chair and started to weep. I almost did too!

Before I could stop myself, I heard myself suggest that she go into her nearest children's hospital and read to the children in the burns unit. As Bella wept I inwardly berated myself for the insensitivity of suggesting such a dreadful thing to someone who, presumably, had only weeks to live.

When she was ready I passed her some tissues and, between sobs, Bella told me that the greatest grief and sadness in her life was the fact that she had never had children. She had ached to have them but her husband, who was several years older than she was, had never wanted to have a family. She thought the idea of reading quietly to children who were suffering would be wonderful therapy for her.

The third suggestion made no sense to me, but on the strength of Bella's previous response, I decided to proceed. I told her that it might be more helpful for her to forget about her meditation practice and instead listen to the slow movement of the *Double Violin Concerto in D Minor* by Bach each day as if she had never heard it before.

Again Bella's eyes welled up with tears that overflowed and poured down her cheeks. We sat for some time in silence and then she told me this story.

When she was a young child she had particularly loved the violin. Bella's father used to play to her and as soon as she was old enough she had been given a violin of her own and had begun lessons with him. She had been a gifted violinist and had studied the instrument for many years, playing in several quartets, trios and orchestras until she met her husband, who hated the violin. Bella had gradually resigned from the musical activities she was involved in and finally ceased to play at all. The last piece of music she had been perfecting was the very concerto I had suggested she listen to.

Bella and I sat for some time in silence and enjoyed the sense of being at one together. I cannot describe how special these moments are to me. There's a sense of having journeyed together into a deep and rarely visited place and, having retrieved a treasure which resided there, we return refreshed, renewed and able to feel more alive than before.

By releasing the past we're more easily able to enjoy the present and begin to give love and attention to others. Bella's whole posture and demeanour had changed and she looked radiant, beautiful and very much at peace with herself. When I told her so, her smile reflected those qualities and more.

Several beautiful cards arrived from Bella over the ensuing months. Each one described the joy and satisfaction she received from her work with the children in the burns unit. She would usually have a PS at the end of the card saying something like, 'Tumours still there but not bothering me.' A year later she was organising other women to go into the hospital to continue her work. She died very peacefully in her garden chair, eighteen months after our first and only meeting.

BILL

Many people, when faced with illness, must give up work. And they often find they have, in part, identified who they are by what they do in the workplace. This stripping away of identity can be very painful as we question our value to ourselves and to society.

Bill's salvation was in his ready willingness to help others in a very practical way. Bill was a regular member of our support group for people with HIV/AIDS. He had been attending the groups for four or five years. During that time he had journeyed with many of the participants through their own difficulties and illnesses, and many, many had died. Bill had been unable to work for some time because of his health and that eventually necessitated him moving back to his parents' home as he could no longer afford the rent on his flat. He also began to feel more and more dependent on the company of others – most find the long and tedious journey of fluctuating health very hard to bear alone.

Bill's parents lived in a smaller city some distance from Sydney and, though they loved him dearly, the arrangement was not a happy one. Bill was removed from his group of friends and from the satisfaction, purpose and sense of identity his work had provided. His parents came from a Latvian culture far removed from the one Bill had created for himself. One of the only outlets for Bill was coming to Sydney each week by train to the support group I facilitated.

Over the last few months Bill had had some frightening episodes with dementia, sometimes finding himself in a supermarket or street with no idea who he was, where he was going or where his home was. He began to lose confidence in himself at an alarming rate. His identity seemed to be slipping away from him and each day brought new and unwanted problems with his memory and general vagueness. He found his parents' lifestyle and company increasingly difficult to cope with. His mother was always trying to get him to eat, and his father tried to involve him in his handyman activities which didn't interest Bill at all. As his home situation deteriorated he became more and more unhappy with his living arrangements. His parents were forever encouraging him to have early nights and were doing their best to take care of their 'little boy'. He loved them dearly, but the more they treated him like a child, the more desperate he became.

Bill would share his concerns, frustrations and fears each week in the group. He became depressed and dispirited and missed a couple of sessions. Others in the group telephoned him to encourage him not to lose heart and to let him know they were thinking of him.

One day Bill walked into the support group room with a spring in his step and a sparkle in his eye. He told us that he'd moved out of home after seeing an advertisement for a live-in carer for schizophrenics in a community housing project. His self-esteem improved immediately because he was now of use to others. He would take them shopping and on other activities and help to educate them about functioning in the community. When he was feeling vague or a bit lost himself, they would take care of him. This proved to be a saving grace for him as he had his independence, self-esteem and a sense of worth and identity once more. Out of his own need and struggle for peace and contentment, Bill came up with a solution that was tailor-made for him.

Bill showed enormous courage in overcoming his frustration, lack of self-esteem and fear. He was able to see beyond his own struggles with dementia to the problems of those faced by people with schizophrenia. Peace comes to us in many ways and Bill's self-worth was re-established by his unstinting support of others. The glory in his story is that when he was lost himself, it gave his charges the opportunity to help him. Healing for all.

JENNY

Rituals that help us deal with our feelings of loss, sadness and grief can be potent tools to finding resolution. Without resolution, these emotions can continue to destroy our peace and undermine our efforts to move forward with our lives. I believe that this lack of resolution can also undermine our body's efforts to heal or to progress to another stage of physical growth.

Sarah brought her very shy twelve-year-old daughter to see me. Jenny was slowly recovering from chronic fatigue syndrome which she had developed when she was nine after a bout of glandular fever. She had had three years of fluctuating health and wasn't doing particularly well at school because she was only attending for half days. She took prescribed medication every night to get to sleep and had become completely dependent on it. She'd lie awake for hours if she didn't take her sedative. She was fairly picky about what she'd eat and her appetite was small. Jenny had many allergies and was pale and small for her age. Her teachers complained that she was withdrawn at school and found it difficult to make friends.

Like Emma, Jenny was loathe to talk to me, and I knew it would take a little while for her to trust me. I asked her mother to tell me about the time Jenny had glandular fever, then I would check out the story with Jenny herself later. The story unfolded.

At the time of her glandular fever, Jenny's adored nanna was receiving treatment for cancer. Because of the chemotherapy her grandmother was undergoing, her immune system was depressed and she was told not to get close to Jenny because she might pick up the child's infection. When Nanna visited, she always came to Jenny's door to talk and blow kisses.

Finally Nanna entered hospital for the last time. When she had said her goodbyes to Jenny and blown her kisses from the doorway, she'd told her she was getting better. And Jenny believed her.

Throughout this story, Jenny remained silent and I wondered if she would be able to fill in some of the details from her own perspective.

I told Jenny a story about my own grandmother as a way of encouraging her to talk. Little did I know that the story I told would have such an immediate and powerful effect.

I adored my grandmother who was a loving and spirited woman. She was also one of the most enthusiastic and irreverent people I have ever been blessed to know. In her sixties she even married a minister on condition that he never mention religion in the house! I told Jenny that when I was a young child, Granny and I would go for walks around the block in our suburb. She would always take a basket and a pair of secateurs, and if any plant took her eye, she would snip off a cutting and place it into the basket. I thought this was terribly daring. Sometimes, if the plant was over a fence, Granny, undaunted, would lean over, or even enter the property if she thought no one was home, and relieve the owners of their greenery. I used to be mortified at her naughtiness and expect the police to arrive at any moment. Jenny's eyes had begun to sparkle and enlarge and she spoke for the first time saying, 'My nanna used to do that too!'

I continued, telling Jenny that my granny had a special smell about her and that I loved to visit her home which was dark, cool and inviting. I loved the sound of the water spattering onto the leaves outside the window when Granny set the hose to spray her beloved plants at the end of the day. These all seemed to be things Jenny could relate to and she told me somewhat forlornly that she missed the smell of her nanna.

I asked her about her nanna's death and how she found out that she had died. Jenny said that when the phone call came to say Nanna had died, she only heard that the news was bad. She surmised that her grandmother had died, though no-one actually told her directly.

The relationship Jenny and her nanna had shared was a powerful one, and she was sad she had never said goodbye and that in those last weeks she couldn't even hug or kiss her. She was bewildered by illness, death, loss and unacknowledged grief.

With Jenny's hesitant and tearful cooperation we discussed how she felt about illness, cancer, not being told directly about her nanna's death, not having the opportunity to say goodbye. Then, with more enthusiasm and joy, she spoke of what she loved and missed about her grandmother.

Together we mapped out a plan. Firstly I reassured Jenny that lots of people felt the way she did, and that even adults have a hard time talking about people who have died because they feel the hurt inside when they do.

I suggested she and her mother create a ritual out of going to bed, which would include a warm bath, being wrapped in a rainbow and then sending another rainbow from her heart to wherever Nanna was.

I suggested that when Jenny was snuggled down with her eyes closed and ready for sleep, Sarah could run her hand lightly over the whole of Jenny's body and ask her to imagine that she was wrapping her in a cloud of red, the colour of tomatoes and postboxes. Sarah could continue running her hand softly over her body and ask Jenny to imagine that she was being wrapped in a cloud of orange, the colour of nasturtiums and oranges. Then yellow, the colour of daffodils and sunshine; and green, the colour of spring leaves and grass. Then blue, the colour of the sky; violet, the colour of the flower violet; and indigo, the colour of the night sky. At the end Sarah could place her hand over Jenny's heart and ask her to imagine as vividly as possible a rainbow which started in her heart and then came out through the air to Sarah's heart. This rainbow would keep them connected all through the night. Jenny could then send another rainbow from her heart to wherever Nanna was now.

Because she had formed the habit of taking sleeping medication and was afraid to stop, I prescribed a herbal formula to be taken in addition to her usual medication. This formula is very good for calming down restlessness in the body and tends to soothe and relax. I reassured her that she could sleep with the light on until she was an old lady if she wanted. Once Jenny was confident our plan was working, she could start taking her sedative medication on alternate nights. Then, after a period of weeks, when she felt ready, she could stop it altogether. After that she could begin reducing the herbal formula in the same way. When she was ready to settle for sleep she could play one of my guided imagery tapes – 'Dolphin Magic', a favourite of many children.

I also suggested that Jenny might like to make a special present for her nanna. I could tell this immediately captured her attention and curiosity. Her present could consist of a letter telling her nanna how much she loved her and what she missed about her. It could perhaps contain a story of a favourite time they'd spent together, or an occasion of love or laughter; she might even like to include some drawings or a special photograph of her and her nanna together, or some trinket they had both enjoyed. All this, I suggested, could be placed inside a covered shoe box and tied with ribbons of her nanna's favourite colours. By now Jenny looked animated at the prospect of her 'secret' present to Nanna.

I then suggested she and her mother drive to a nursery and Jenny choose a tree or rosebush to plant in the garden, perhaps outside her bedroom window. At the base of this tree she could bury her present. Then Jenny could shovel in the earth and this would be Nanna's tree, a place where Jenny could always come and have a chat to her grandmother or send her rainbows. Over the years she could watch it grow as her love for her nanna continued to grow.

Sarah telephoned me three weeks later to tell me that Jenny was off all medication, had become much happier and, according to her teachers, was now quite a chatterbox in class. She was sleeping soundly all night with the light off and with no need of either the herbal or prescribed sedative. I saw her about two months after our initial conversation and she had colour in her cheeks and was eating a full diet and attending school for five full days once more.

Six months later I saw Jenny in the street. She was very self-assured and a welcoming smile came readily to her face. She had grown considerably since we met and had clearly entered puberty. We hugged and I asked her if she had ever made that present for her nanna or planted a remembrance tree. Her reply surprised and delighted me. 'No, I haven't,' she said, 'but I know I can.'

Jenny had felt angry, abandoned, confused and sad at her nanna's death. Feelings are not just states of mind. We produce chemicals in our brain in accordance with how we feel. The chemicals of anger, abandonment, confusion and sadness can affect our health if we neglect to find healing and resolution for them. When we cry, talk, write, scream, draw, plant, hear stories, meditate or do whatever we need to do in order to give expression to our feelings, we find peace and resolution. In this way, the events which have caused us pain can become part of our history rather than something which continues to impede our ability to live well now.

Jenny needed permission to feel the emotions she was experiencing. She also needed to understand her feelings and hear acknowledgement from someone that her relationship with her grandmother was precious and that though her nanna was dead, her love for her would continue and perhaps even deepen throughout her life.

Children are often bewildered by the strength and depth of feelings they haven't experienced before. They need reassurance from those around them that these feelings are understandable and that it is alright for them to feel so intensely. Sometimes, if the rest of the family is grieving, the child's feelings may be overlooked. If we neglect to grieve, or stop our grieving, it waits for us to give it the time and space it deserves.

I thought I had grieved long and healthily over Brenden's death until fourteen years later I visited Kathmandu for the first time. The experience amazed and overwhelmed me.

My partner Wendie and I were in India for a conference on women and spirituality and had decided to continue on and visit Nepal. There was so much mystery surrounding Brenden's death and, though I knew the lapse in time would make finding out any details virtually impossible, I needed to walk the same streets, smell the air and feel the atmosphere of the city where he had spent his last days. I had faxed ahead to the British Embassy, who had arranged Brenden's cremation, telling them of my visit.

As our plane began its descent I felt a great well of emotion bubble up inside me. I swallowed the lump in my throat and made myself busy with our landing preparations. I was on holiday – surely this wasn't going to turn into some sort of cathartic event! The emotions surfaced time and again over the next few days. Wendie was wonderfully supportive and encouraging and let me weep whenever I needed to.

Brenden had gone to the British Embassy to seek assistance for his depression and the staff had been very kind to him. They had suggested he stay in a hotel opposite the embassy as they had a function on that evening. They'd asked him to return first thing the next morning and they would help him then. He never saw the dawning of that morning.

The day I entered the grounds of the embassy I lost all control and sobbed like a lost soul. I found it astounding that so many uncried tears still remained and it reminded me of the words a mother whose daughter had died of AIDS had used to describe her grief.

'My grief is like the rain,' she said. 'Some days it is just a few spatters against the window. Other times it's a steady drizzle all day. And on others it's an absolute downpour.'

MICHAEL

In our support groups we're given the opportunity to air our fears, angers and apprehensions and perhaps gain another perspective. Nothing is more healing than to laugh at something which was once fearful to us but which now has no power over us. There's a silent permission permeating the group which allows for free expression of whatever emotions are being experienced, be they grief, panic, anger, frustration, depression, regret, sadness, joy, love, fear, guilt, powerlessness or anything else.

There's no agenda for the groups. We don't set out to talk about any particular subject. Each session is unique and special in its own way. All our groups are open so new members are always welcome. We find people cannot always commit themselves to being there every week because of treatments or other responsibilities. And not everyone wants to come every week. Many of our participants have to travel great distances to experience this support. Each week in our groups in Bundanoon we have people who travel from Sydney, Canberra, Wollongong and the Blue Mountains.

Michael was a member of our Monday group a few years ago when it was based in Sydney. He used to travel down from the Blue Mountains to the group each week. He was always very well dressed and even though he was only thirty-four, his illness meant he had to walk with a cane. He was much loved by the group because of his wicked sense of humour and his loving compassion for others.

On one particular Monday he told us he needed to go for a certain treatment immediately after the group. This treatment always made him terribly sick for three days afterwards and he wasn't looking forward to it at all as he was already feeling frail. The group assured him they'd be sending lots of love and rainbows to him in the next few days. Just before he left he commented on how much he loved gardenias. There were half a dozen left in the garden and I picked them for him.

When he arrived at the hospital, he was given the same dosage of drugs he had received in his previous treatment. However, he was sixteen kilos *lighter* this time and ended up, due to the hospital's failure to take this into account, receiving quite an overdose. He managed to get home to his apartment in the city where he collapsed on the floor inside the front door. His friends had expected him to return to his Blue Mountains home and so his absence wasn't noticed. Michael wasn't discovered for two days.

The following Monday, very much the worse for wear, Michael told us of his ordeal. 'I lay on the floor and I couldn't move. I thought I was dying and I felt so afraid, but there was the smell of gardenias. The pain was indescribable and I felt so alone, but there were flashes of rainbows and moments of warmth when I knew I was being loved. In this way, remembering love, rainbows and gardenias, I survived until help arrived.'

Sometimes we can't change what happens to us, but we can join together to give strength and comfort to one another.

For me, the sending of rainbows is the essence of prayer. We visualise the person and see them healed and whole and at peace. When we extend our love and peace to them we know that its presence will bring comfort, hope and strength.

You might like to join us in a daily ritual that we've created in order to reach out in love and support of one another. This ritual has spread through several internet support groups and is now practised by thousands of people around the world.

Each afternoon at four o'clock we spend two minutes centering ourselves by bringing all our awareness into the present moment. We do this by connecting our awareness with the senses of the body, feeling our weight and posture, the touch of our clothing and the air against our skin. We listen to all the sounds within and outside the room we're in and we let our breathing be soft and easy. Then we visualise that we're sitting under one end of a bright and beautiful rainbow, and all the iridescent colours surround and envelop us. We take a moment to breathe in our favourite colours and then we extend the other end of the rainbow out through the ceiling to all who are in need of healing. We visualise our love and blessings flowing out across those rainbows to wherever they're needed.

Rainbows bypass the mind and speak to the heart. They are symbols of magic and can serve as a reminder of the promise of hope. They are the bridge between the worlds of darkness and light, and by heeding their message we can create an environment for healing within ourselves and those whom our lives touch.

GRAHAM

The problem with many of our unpleasant feelings is that we *resist* them. Then we have to *suppress* them in order to continue functioning 'normally'. We are often scared of our feelings because of their intensity, or we judge the ones that we don't like as being less important, or bad, compared to our happier ones. This can lead to a dislocation between how we feel and what we present to the world outside.

Many people think that if they've suppressed the unpleasant memory of some past event, they will not have to feel the feelings associated with it. However, these feelings continue to reside within us and undermine our peace. Once expressed we are free of their negative effect within us, though this can take a long time and a lot of effort.

A lot of people make the mistake of thinking that if

we feel our fear, or any other feelings associated with our thoughts, then that is negative. For instance, if we have a life-threatening illness and we think about dying, our feelings about dying will surface also. Many people will then suggest that those thoughts are negative and should be abolished. What nonsense! I used to think, 'If I think about dying, then maybe I'm programming myself that it is OK to die and it's *not* OK.' I would then be terrified of letting my thoughts wander in that direction, believing that I might somehow speed up the process.

It was a major turning point for me when I dragged death out of the corner, placed it firmly in the centre of the room and let myself think and feel my way through the issues around my death and dying. I became friends with my feelings rather than fearing them. This enabled me to move beyond those feelings, then I was ready to really live *today.*

Meditation can be one of the most effective ways in which we can begin to address these feelings and allow them expression. Through meditation we find a rock-solid place of peace within ourselves that is beyond the fear, beyond the pain, beyond all thought and all feeling; a place in which we know that the essence of our being is love.

Paradoxically, to acknowledge that I am afraid, for instance, and give myself permission to feel afraid is the first step towards being released from fear. Meditation gives us the opportunity to *witness* the fear without becoming overwhelmed by it.

Gradually we come to realise that these are only feelings and that they aren't the sum total of who we are.

Graham had HIV and was finding the uncertainty of the future and the difficulties of the present too much to bear. The destruction of his immune system had led to damaged eyesight, massive weight loss, pneumonia, thrombocytopenia and the removal of his spleen, skin irritations, sinus problems and unrelenting diarrhoea.

Graham had had little time to take on board the reality of his HIV before his body started to manifest all these unwanted symptoms. He struggled to maintain a sense of normality, but his body made more and more demands of him that he found increasingly difficult to ignore.

Graham held a senior position in the firm that he worked for and had several staff within his division. He would go to extraordinary lengths to make sure that no-one at work knew of his suffering. He was unsure of how his staff would react to his HIV diagnosis and felt that the longer he could conceal his disease the better. To convince the people he worked with that all was well, he'd made up stories about needing to lose weight, age affecting his eyesight, tummy upsets from something he ate, and so on. This terrible double life alienated him from any of the support he might have received had he been more open and honest, but he was unsure how to unravel the mess he had got himself into.

Graham began coming to our weekly support groups and instantly relaxed as he found others shared his experiences and the myriad feelings which accompanied them. He loved meditation as it complemented his spiritual beliefs and deepened his connection with his religion.

As the months passed, Graham was able to include

more and more of his friends and work associates in the knowledge of his diagnosis, and was delighted and touched by the amount of support which was readily extended to him.

On one occasion Graham came to the group quite animated. He told us this story. He had sat at his desk with tears rolling down his cheeks. His staff had anxiously asked, 'Graham, whatever's the matter?'

He replied, 'I'm just not coping!'

At lunch time he had gone out to order his sandwich from the local shop and Guiseppe, the shopkeeper, had said to him: 'Graham, you're crying. What's wrong?'

'I'm just not coping,' he had replied.

He told the support group: 'I've spent all my life coping. It's a wonderful relief to let go and not cope.'

The experience of life-threatening illness, or any crisis for that matter, can allow us to become authentic. Instead of always trying to measure up to our own or other people's expectations we can simply become *real* without having to hide bits of ourself from ourselves or others.

Many of us are afraid of our feelings and yet to give them expression is enormously healthy. With the help of meditation we can follow three simple steps.

1. First we identify or acknowledge the feeling.
2. Then we give ourselves permission to feel that way.
3. Then we simply feel the feeling.

For instance, this might be how it was for Graham.

1. This is how it feels to be me, Graham, not coping.

2. It's OK for me not to cope.
3. This is how not coping feels to me.

Paradoxically that *is* coping. Not coping might mean weeping, pulling the doona over your head, screaming or going for a walk along the beach.

If we follow these three simple steps, we are more easily able to deal with our feelings. Give yourself whole-hearted permission to not cope. You might want to put some constraints around not coping. 'I give myself whole-hearted permission to not cope until two o'clock this afternoon. Then I'll have a shower, get dressed and go and face the world again, but up until then, count me out!'

Likewise with fear. Much of my life was spent trying not to feel fear. I had to expend enormous amounts of energy pretending to be positive in order to convince myself and everyone else that I had no fear. In this way, fear had me completely trapped. Once I was able to bring the fear out into the light of day, its enormous power vanished. The fastest way out of feelings is through them.

Peace is not a wishy-washy state of passive acceptance. It's a dynamic state in which we embrace whatever is going on in our lives. If we feel anger, fear, despair, panic, outrage, resentment or anything else, we bring it out in the open, acknowledge it, express it and then are more easily able to let go of it. This is what peace is about. It's not about sitting on a hotbed of emotions hoping or pretending they don't exist. Give them your whole-hearted permission to come out into the light, to be expressed and understood.

Many people are afraid to express how they feel to someone else because they fear ridicule or abuse of the trust they've extended. It's important to be respectful of our feelings and to choose wisely those with whom we seek to share our vulnerability.

MARIA

It can be confusing sometimes if we think that healing is about keeping people alive. It is really about a deeper healing, the healing of our spirit. Rather than thinking we're simply bodies that need attention, we need to focus on the whole of an individual and make the spiritual healing of that person our primary goal.

We are each here to find our own healing and the events of our lives can become the catalyst by which we find that profound healing.

One Wednesday afternoon brought a call from a distraught mother whose fourteen-year-old daughter, Maria, was struggling with the side effects of chemotherapy. Her oncologist had referred her to me because Maria wanted to discontinue her treatment and he felt that some counselling might help her cope more effectively.

Maria had a lymphoma which her treatment had

done little to arrest. One of the tumours affected the spinal cord in her neck and she was beginning to notice weakness and tingling in both her arms and legs. She only came twice to my rooms before paralysis set in and made it impossible for her to travel to see me.

The disease had moved very quickly and left Maria's family devastated. They were of Italian background and had only arrived in Australia eighteen months before Maria's diagnosis. Her parents, Carla and Tony, had worked hard to establish a business and to integrate into a new culture in order to create a home and lifestyle for themselves and their only child.

When Maria began to experience unrelenting headaches they initially put it down to stress as she struggled with her studies in a new language. Before long, however, it became obvious that something more serious was wrong.

To negotiate the hospital system and medical language is a challenge for most people, let alone those for whom English is a second language. Both Carla and Tony attended all of Maria's appointments and treatments even though this created a financial strain as they spent less time working in their business. They owned a corner shop which relied solely on the three of them to manage.

As settling into Australia had been their first priority, they had not formed any close friendships and had no family in the city in which they lived. Tony's sister, Nerida, lived in Melbourne and was able to give only limited support as she too was working hard at creating a new life for her family.

Carla, Tony and Maria formed a close-knit family unit dependent on one another but no-one else. Maria had made some friends at school, but because of her illness only one of them had continued to visit. Indra was shy and quiet, yet she enjoyed coming to Maria's home each week to talk about the students at school and their activities. Indra had recently emigrated to Australia from Indonesia and the two girls had formed a bond based upon their struggles to adjust to a new country, culture and language. Maria tried to keep up with her school work but it quickly became a frustrating task that was beyond her. Her mother was unable to assist her as her English wasn't good enough, and Indra's visits were times of conversation rather than study.

Carla and Tony accompanied Maria into the consultation room the first time she came to see me. It quickly became apparent that they were sizing me up to see if they felt comfortable having me involved with their precious daughter; having passed this test, Maria and I spent the time alone together on subsequent visits.

Maria's family held very strong Catholic beliefs which gave them a great deal of comfort. Though much in this new country was strange to them and the hospital system was intimidating, they had trust in Maria's doctors whom they felt had her best interests at heart. As it became clear that the treatments were failing to help Maria, Tony became withdrawn and moody, leaving most of the physical care of Maria to her mother. He felt helpless against this life-threatening intruder which had the power to rob him of just about everything he held dear and which made a mockery of his efforts to create a new life for his family. He was used to taking care of his family and solving any problems they might have. It was the first time he had been confronted with his inability to change what *is*.

Tony found it increasingly difficult even to look at Maria without his eyes brimming with tears. As her paralysis increased, Tony spent more and more time in the shop, leaving before she awoke and coming home long after she was asleep. The shop was open seven days a week, and although Maria understood that she broke his heart, she missed his company and the way he used to ruffle her hair and call her his angel.

Many of Tony's customers were also newcomers to Australia and the word quickly got around of the family's unfolding tragedy. Maria had served many of them in the shop and they remembered her fondly as not only a beautiful young girl but one whose heart was good. They began to drop in gifts for her at the shop and always enquired about how things were going. Tony initially fobbed off these enquiries, feeling that he shouldn't impose his personal problems on his business life; he seemed to feel too that Maria's illness was somehow a reflection on his ability to take care of his family.

Occasionally one of his customers would bring in a cooked meal for Carla to reheat. She was able to accept this with gratitude far more readily than Tony, who again felt it was a sign of weakness that they needed help.

Maria had deduced that her treatment was ineffective and she wanted to stop the weekly visits to the hospital. She now needed to be carried to the car and had to rely on a wheelchair at the hospital. She felt that this was distressing and disruptive for her family, that it created a financial strain and the treatment made her feel wretched.

With her parents absent Maria spoke with dignity and courage about her impending death, and her main concerns centred around how her parents would cope without her. She had often served as the go-between for them as her English was better than theirs. She had actually understood more about the seriousness of her disease than her parents and felt it a burden to have to reassure them when she knew that her disease was little affected by the treatment.

In our second session together she said simply, 'I know I'm going to die, but how will my parents cope?'

Her words hung in the air unanswered. I sat close beside her and, holding one another, she wept quietly while I felt my heart break with the sadness that all children and parents face with the impending death of a child.

When I spoke with Maria's oncologist about her treatment he confirmed that it wasn't helping her but that Maria's father had wanted to continue it if there was any hope at all. I suspected that some of their confusion was due to the language barrier and that they had chosen to hear only what was hopeful. Maria's oncologist was in agreement about discontinuing her treatment and decided to speak with her parents alone with an interpreter.

After this visit to the oncologist both Tony and Carla were able to cry and comfort one another and Carla became determined to care for Maria at home herself.

She refused any community nursing help and spent all day, every day attending to Maria's needs, believing that no-one could care for her in quite the same way as she could. It was only during my visit to their home or when Nerida was able to stay a few days that Carla had any respite.

Tony felt that ceasing Maria's treatment gave him permission to face, for the first time, his growing hopelessness and this allowed him to focus on what he could do to show Maria how enormously he loved her.

Maria showed an unusual depth of understanding about meditation and each time I visited her we would practise together. In between my visit to her home each week she would practise at least three times daily with one of the relaxation tapes I had made. Maria felt that it gave her a safe place to retreat to when the sensations in her lifeless limbs became irritating. She experienced a lot of restlessness in her arms and legs but, because she could not move them, could find little relief.

One of the pictures hanging in my office had attracted Maria and seemed to mean a great deal to her. It was of a pathway that led through gnarled trees to a beautiful sunrise. The sun wasn't actually visible, but the soft glowing light gave a strong impression of the coming dawn. She told me that keeping this image in her mind helped her to enter a meditative state. She would imagine that she was moving down the path and that each of the gnarled trees was a different part of her life or her body that she wanted to let go. Her aim was to stand in the clearing beyond the trees where she could see and feel the light without any distraction. When she could imagine that strongly, she would feel deeply content and at peace.

I decided that the painting belonged to Maria. When I gave it to her, her whole face lit up with joy and peace. It was hung on her bedroom wall so she could see it as she lay in her bed, and later, when she could no longer move her head, it was hung on the ceiling.

The next time I visited Maria she was completely paralysed. Carla was finding the physical care of her more demanding and there were complications such as severe constipation and incontinence. It is a challenge to find peace when your body is so distressed. Her appetite was still quite good and she wasn't particularly wasted. The tone of Maria's bowel was being affected by the tumours in her spine and it was obvious that Carla was beyond coping without professional palliative expertise. When Carla understood that Maria could be made more comfortable if she allowed the nurses to help, she gave way. I arranged for an Italian-speaking palliative care nurse to come to their home, and Carla and Maria took to Philomena immediately. Each day Philomena would drop in to help wash and change Maria and answer any questions Carla might have about her physical care.

Maria was finding swallowing difficult and she was afraid of choking on her food, even though Carla made sure everything was soft and easy to manage. She ate less and less and seemed to drift into a peaceful world of her own, emerging from time to time to say something loving and supportive to her parents or to request a drink or to be moved.

I was amazed by Maria's ability to adapt to so many losses with such good grace. She had been a beautiful girl just entering into young womanhood and here she lay inert and incontinent without the least trace of bitterness or depression.

Tony began spending more and more time with his daughter now. At first, he made sure that he was home in time to ruffle her hair and to kiss her goodnight. Then he started reading her Italian folk stories and fairy tales. Sometimes he'd tell her the story of their life in Italy and their journey to a new land and a new life. They would often drift off to sleep together, she in her bed and Tony in the armchair pulled up beside her. Sometimes, sitting by her as she slept and stroking her brow gently so as not to wake her, he'd weep.

My last visit to Maria was on a cold and drizzly Saturday morning. The atmosphere in the house was unmistakable. There was an air of solemnity: candles had been lit and Nerida and Carla chanted prayers while Maria slept. She had barely been conscious in the previous twenty-four hours. Her room was full of flowers from Tony's customers, and above her bed on the ceiling were pictures of saints, her family, myself and the painting that had once hung in my office. I was deeply moved to be included in what she called her 'healing team'.

After hugging Carla, Nerida and Tony, I bent to kiss Maria's forehead. She awoke a moment later and I turned her head towards me so that our eyes could meet. I was taken aback by the sparkle in her eyes. There seemed so much joy and peace dancing there as she said to me, 'Petrea, how can this be dying when I feel so alive inside?'

Maria's family and I sat with this mystery until she drifted into unconsciousness and, finally, with an almost imperceptible sigh, left us.

Carla and Tony were deeply touched by the love and support they received from the many people they had first met as customers in their shop but with whom, through Maria's illness, they had since forged friendships that continued to sustain them. At Maria's funeral the church was filled with these new-found friends. Tony and Carla struggled with their grief but no longer felt like strangers in a new land. Carla wept with the women who continued to drop in for a cuppa or to bring them meals. Together they poured over photographs and talked of Maria's past accomplishments and talents. The men supported Tony in different ways, inviting him to go fishing or occasionally helping him unload heavy boxes at his shop. During these activities Tony's grief was accepted and accommodated. Carla and Tony had a community on which they knew they could rely, because friendships formed in the midst of tragedy are already tested by adversity.

It isn't uncommon for people moving towards death to experience a reality in which, in complete contrast to what's happening in their bodies, they find a strength and depth of aliveness rarely experienced by those even in excellent health. Their peace and contentment is not dictated by their achievements or by what is happening to their bodies. They can find a place of indestructible peace beyond their physical suffering.

This is not only true for those who are ill but is often true for their loved ones too. I've witnessed the tremendous love and tenderness shown by a husband whose wife lay terribly disfigured and ravaged by her disease. Stroking her lovingly, he spoke tenderly of her great beauty. Oblivious to the smells, sounds or ugliness that her disease had produced, he saw only the beauty that had attracted him to her in the first place.

The human spirit has the capacity to find love and experience a deep sense of oneness with another person even in the midst of the most painful suffering. It is as if the illness strips away every layer that separates the deep joining of spirits. However, it takes a great willingness to allow this to unfold for each person rails against the disease in their unique ways.

More often than not it is the parents who need support and understanding as they take on the enormity of the tragedy of losing a child. It isn't so much a matter of giving them any advice as listening to their pain as they struggle to accept the reality of their loss and the misery of a future without one they hold so dear. With love and support the healing of such misery is possible, though the darkness of grief assails us in every moment. Life *does* continue even though, initially, we might only be able to go through the motions of living. The sharing of tears and the retelling of our story are essentials in this healing process. With each telling we move closer to healing, and gradually a glimmer of light appears and we find the strength within ourselves to give life our full commitment once more.

CHARLIE

Some years ago I was invited to America to work with Dr Jerry Jampolsky, a psychiatrist who specialised in working with children with life-threatening illnesses. It seemed an invaluable opportunity to work alongside someone I respected so much and who could answer many of my questions about how most effectively to help sick children. I was to spend two weeks with Jerry. Everything was geared to this – flights booked and paid for, accommodation organised and arrangements made to cope with my growing practice in my absence.

Then I met Charlie.

Charlie was nine years old and had been undergoing treatment for cancer for some months. His cancer had progressed to the point where he was very weak. His family was absolutely devoted to him and was nursing him at home. His bed had been set up in the family room and Charlie was the centre of all that happened in the house. His mother, Sally, had asked me in to help Charlie with his visualisation practices. He and I liked each other immediately. He had developed a very complex visualisation which involved a beautiful white horse who was his friend and wise companion, a forest and an army of little white-jacketed men who sprayed the weeds growing in this forest. This signified to him the chemotherapy killing off the cancerous growths in his body.

I told Charlie and his family about my trip to America in five weeks' time. When I told Charlie why I was going away and asked him how he felt about my going, he closed his eyes and, after a little time, replied: 'There are going to be a lot of children like me in your life. I think you'd better go and get your questions answered.'

Over the ensuing weeks I became deeply involved with the whole family. Charlie was terribly ill and I offered what support I could. Every now and again I'd remind Charlie of my increasingly imminent departure. Each time, he would simply acknowledge that he knew I was about to go. His parents had supported my decision to go but had also offered to reimburse any cancellation costs should I decide to stay. I wasn't feeling at all happy about leaving as my instinct was to stay.

The day finally came when I was due to fly out of Australia. I stopped by Charlie's home on the way to the airport to say goodbye. Charlie was sound asleep. His family left me alone with him and I sat by his bed with my own sad thoughts. I said my goodbyes to Charlie silently in my heart and then suddenly had a profound realisation that Charlie knew the answers to the questions I had planned to ask Jerry Jampolsky. I also knew that Charlie's answers would involve heart-breaking suffering, and would not be nearly as pleasant as my proposed trip. Nevertheless, there was no doubt in my mind that I should stay.

By listening to Charlie's and my unspoken needs I learned what was going on under the surface. *Really* listening is the most important thing that anyone can bring to any situation dealing with the sensitive issues of others. I could not have understood anything more precious had I gone to America and worked with Jerry. I knew the answers I'd receive from Charlie wouldn't be theoretical ones but would be borne out of the experience of our united suffering.

As I had already scheduled two weeks out of my diary, I offered to move in with Charlie and his family to devote myself full-time to being of practical assistance to them. Charlie's parents were grateful for the added support and we grew closer as each day presented its challenges and difficulties.

We massaged Charlie's feet, head and hands, watched 'Fawlty Towers' videos and read Roald Dahl books. Their home was filled with love, laughter, tears, endless cups of tea and visits from friends and extended family. The family's two adored dogs were Charlie's constant companions and it was wonderful to see how sensitive they were to his increasing frailty. In the midst of the hubbub of family life the dogs often helped to create a little oasis of peace around Charlie.

In his last few months Charlie suffered excruciating pain which his doctors struggled to control. To the family's lasting horror and grief, his pain, despite modern medicine's best efforts and huge doses of morphine, wasn't brought under adequate control. He suffered awful spasms of breakthrough pain which were unpredictable and increasingly frequent. He would cry and moan and close his eyes and lie pale and exhausted once the spasm had passed. To be confronted by our own helplessness and powerlessness to stop the pain in someone we love is surely one of the greatest trials of all. I was tempted at times to leave Charlie's bedside simply because it was hard to be around so much pain, especially in one as young as he. However, that would have been little help to Charlie and even less to his family. From Charlie I gained the courage to face the pain of my own powerlessness and he taught me that the willingness simply to stick around and share the journey is a comfort in itself.

Through Charlie I began to see that the level to which I'm willing to experience my own pain is the level to which I'm able to be with someone else who's in pain. If I refuse to face the pain of my own suffering, then most assuredly I'll stop the other person from confronting me with theirs, perhaps through changing my body posture or through the questions I ask, or neglect to ask, or the comments I make. I could so easily have made an excuse to leave Charlie and his family to attend to some other distraction.

Many of us make excuses for not phoning or visiting someone whose problems we find difficult, overwhelming or too confronting. We all struggle at times with the fear that we will say the wrong thing or simply find no words to say at all. Needless to say, this is of little help to the person whose life has challenged us.

In a difficult or painful situation I've often found that when I can let go needing to *do* something in order to escape my own feelings of powerlessness, then insights begin to appear. When we let go the clutter of our own fears and feelings of helplessness it allows space for our intuition to begin functioning more effectively. Two ideas came to me at this time that each proved to be wonderfully helpful to both Charlie and those of us who loved him.

The first idea concerned the spasms of pain when they initially appeared, coming out of the blue and distressing us all so much. These spasms seemed very similar to a labour contraction, rising and then ebbing in intensity. I asked Charlie if he'd like to try breathing through the pain with me. He was keen to try anything that would help him get through the pain more easily. The next time he had a spasm, I took his hands in mine and, maintaining eye contact throughout, we panted our way through the spasm. This helped us get through the spasm *together* instead of Charlie retreating into himself.

Charlie's sister, Helen, herself only a few years older than her sick brother, asked if she might do this with him too. It seemed to lessen the intensity and duration of the spasms; it might have been that we simply found a way of sharing his pain by participating more deeply in it. I marvelled at the whole family's courage and love and their willingness to meet the challenges we faced daily as we cared for Charlie.

The second idea that occurred to me was that, although Charlie's hand was often held and he was hugged and cuddled, he was never actually held in anyone's arms because of his frailty. We carefully sat Charlie forward so that I could straddle the bed behind him and he could recline in my arms. He loved being held and it helped lessen the intensity of his pain. From then until Charlie died two weeks later he was held in loving arms most of the time. Each member of his family took turns to share this precious time holding Charlie. At night, his family could sleep knowing that he was safe in my arms, or the night nurse's arms, and that we would waken them if there was any need.

Charlie's father Norman initially resisted climbing into bed with his adored son. The thought of being so close to Charlie, especially if he should have an unpredictable spasm of pain, was an enormous challenge. It is an agony to be still and confront our own pain with no distraction. When Norman finally climbed in with Charlie and held him gently in his arms the peaceful look on Charlie's face was something to behold. He drifted off to sleep whilst Norman stroked his son's head and quietly wept.

A few days after my cancelled departure to America, Charlie had a problem which necessitated him being taken to hospital for a few hours. It was a painful and gruelling time for everyone and we came home in the middle of the night exhausted and dispirited. As we settled Charlie back into his own bed he slipped my hand in his and squeezed it as he looked into my eyes and said, 'Thanks for staying.' It wasn't necessary but it was a touching affirmation of my decision to stay with him and weather the storms together.

Charlie died very peacefully in his brother Alexander's arms surrounded by love. His death was a tragedy and he is still missed terribly. But his family can draw comfort from the fact that everything that could be done for him was done and that the loving bonds between them were strong enough to withstand the fires of hell.

SOPHIE

We often believe, mistakenly, that a painful relationship from the past is best forgotten. More often than not, it isn't forgotten: the painful memories are just buried deep down inside ourselves. We may say we don't wish to be reminded of the pain it caused us. But the fact is, it is still causing us pain and we are therefore still in a relationship with that person. The person may no longer be physically present in our lives, but their influence is.

Quite likely, at the time of being hurt, we made some laws about how we would henceforth live our lives. Laws like: 'Never trust men' or 'never trust women'; 'Don't let anyone too close or I'll get hurt'; 'I'd better make sure I get my needs met first, otherwise I'll lose out'; 'Never trust a stranger'; 'Mediocrity is safe', and so on.

Even if the person who hurt us is now dead we

remain in a relationship with them. It is as if there were a rope stretched between that person and ourselves. We are still holding on tight to our end of the rope. When we let go, it sets free a lot of energy previously trapped by the negativity held in that relationship. We may need to let go that rope a hundred times before we're successful in totally forgiving the person, situation or our actions in that situation. We can then learn from the experience and move on. Many people have no desire to forgive those who have hurt them in the past. We sometimes choose to savour our hurts as reasons for us to feel righteous indignation. To let go of the resentment or bitterness also means to let go of the indignation.

By forgiving the past, we can cultivate compassion for others, the compassion we would like to have extended to ourselves. We all make mistakes or make poor choices in our lives. If we recognise those situations as opportunities to learn something new about ourselves or about life, they can become part of our education and we can grow in wisdom because of them.

'Forgiveness is giving up all hope for a better past,' said someone who had finally understood that to rail against the past exhausts us and impedes our progress forward. The past simply *is* as it is. Held resentments and bitterness cause stagnation. When we forgive, we acknowledge that we felt hurt by this person or situation but that it is part of our history and it doesn't have to continue to dominate the present. When we don't forgive, these past hurts and what we've gleaned from them continue to undermine the possibility of peace in the present.

Sophie and her husband, Peter, took an extended holiday, leaving the running of their business in the hands of their partner. On their return they were dismayed to find the woman had mishandled funds deliberately in her favour. The business foundered and it was left to Sophie and Peter to make restitution to a number of creditors. This left them penniless at a time when unemployment was rife and Peter's skills were not in demand. They slowly began putting their life together again, but Sophie in particular, quite understandably, had deep-held feelings of resentment and bitterness toward their former partner. There were also deep feelings of anger and outrage.

About eighteen months after the breakup of the business, Sophie developed breast cancer. For two years she underwent various forms of treatment. The tumours from the primary cancer spread throughout her body, affecting her bones, lungs and liver, and these secondary growths caused her great pain. She blamed her cancer on the stressful time she and Peter had been through. This made her even more angry because she felt that their former partner had deliberately robbed her of her life as well as of their savings.

It was at this point that she joined one of our support groups. She became a regular member and it became obvious that this previous incident still dominated much of her present outlook. Sophie shed many tears in the group over her anger and frustration, and in time it became clear to her that to maintain these feelings held her back from healing and increased her pain. She could see a direct relationship between her pain and the anger and outrage she felt towards their former partner. Whenever she felt a twinge, she would think bitterly that the stress and upset of their business situation had caused her cancer. This in turn made her more distressed and her pain would increase proportionately.

When it became obvious to her that she needed to release the past and forgive her former partner, she sat down to write her a letter. It was a painful and difficult letter to write and she made many attempts before she was finally satisfied with it. She brought the letter to the group to share with us.

Much to everyone's surprise, Sophie had asked the woman to forgive *her* for having held such resentment for all that time. Through the process of looking and relooking at the situation, she had come to realise that it was she, Sophie, who also needed forgiveness. Forgiveness for having held this woman in such a bad light for all this time. Sophie recognised that when we hold resentment and bitterness in our hearts it becomes a poison which harms us. She felt genuine remorse in having held these feelings for so long. She sent the letter away, feeling entirely relieved and saying she didn't need to have a reply as it felt complete for her.

However, very soon, a letter arrived from the woman, pouring out her grief and sadness and asking for forgiveness also. This letter was stained with many splotches from tears. It was amazing to see the transformation which took place in Sophie. Her face softened and she became much more accepting of herself and others. Interestingly enough, her pain level also dropped significantly.

Forgiveness is simple but not necessarily easy. Forgiveness does not mean that we condone the action. We have to work through all the feelings associated with the event before we're ready to accept the fact that a dreadful thing happened and become willing to let it be part of our history rather than something which continues to undermine the peace that is possible in the present moment.

TIM

To work with people who are capable of great violence is a challenge; yet below the surface in every violent person lies a wounded being desperate for understanding, forgiveness or love. Tim embarked upon a remarkable journey in which he healed enormous anger.

One day Tim came to the support group with an axe. He was on his way to his mother's. He had a wild look in his eye and he was trembling. He spoke with hatred about his mother and her attempts to halt the distribution of his late brother's estate. His brother had died of AIDS some six months previously and most of the money was to come to Tim, who also had AIDS. But, Tim's mother wanted the money. She had also wanted sons who were lawyers, bankers or doctors, not, in her words, poofters. His mother had told him she would contest the will so that he would be long dead before its resolution.

Tim had railed against his mother for all the years I had known him. He was desperate for love from her, but she was incapable of giving it. He cajoled, bought her flowers and presents, then he would set her up for failure and remonstrate with her. The family existed in a constant state of manipulation and angst. It was extraordinary to witness his persistence in demanding love from one so incapable of giving it. The more she wanted his conservatism, the more he became reckless, violent and irresponsible.

Tim had turned to prostitution at fifteen, and the frequent knocks at his door were not to enquire about his declining health – which was what he yearned for – but to demand from him something he was no longer able to give. It only served to make him feel more alone, rejected, abandoned and, as a result, angry. Most people were put off by his air of aggression and he found it difficult to make and keep friends.

The support and meditation groups became an oasis for Tim. He allowed us into the turmoil of his sadness, grief and anger. He found friendship, companionship and the understanding of others who also struggled with their family relationships.

Tim attended many of our residential programs in the country. Each time his laughter came a little more spontaneously. Likewise his tears flowed more effortlessly, without the filters of anger and rage. He gradually lost his ferocity.

One of the rituals we shared on these residential programs was the lighting of candles in memory of our many losses and in celebration of the gifts we had received through those losses. In my mind's eye, I can clearly see Tim helping someone even more frail than himself to pick up a candle, light it from the central fire and place it amongst the flowers on the 'altar' where some fifty or more flames flickered.

Tim struggled with the notion of peace. In our groups we often talked of how peace can create the very best of environments for healing within our bodies, minds and spirits. If I taught a forgiveness meditation, Tim would likely say, 'Peace isn't everything!', and yet he ached for resolution and internal harmony.

A year or more before he died, Tim moved to a small government housing apartment. A gay couple who lived upstairs were keen to offer Tim assistance how ever they could. Each evening he would join Ken and Eric for a meal and they often took him out or away for a weekend. Caring for someone who's frail and often irritable and depressed is a challenge for anyone. The boys supported him financially, practically and emotionally in a way I'd only ever seen the closest of families do.

Eric and Ken's love and commitment in caring for their friend was inspiring for those of us who witnessed the transformation which gradually took place within Tim. I have seen many such instances within the gay community of this kind of support being extended. The extraordinary depth of human suffering within this marginalised community has galvanised its members to find and express the purest form of love and compassion to one another.

As Tim became more frail, Ken gave up work to care for him. He cooked for him and kept his apartment clean; he took him daily to the hospital for treatments and drove him wherever he needed to go. Tim continued with the weekly support groups and in time began to see that he was, in fact, enormously loved and cared for – it just didn't come from the source where he had long demanded it. His face became transformed and the hardness went out of it. Occasionally the steely glint and familiar violence would flash through his eyes but would never stay.

When I visited Tim in hospital just before he died, he lay peacefully in Ken's arms. The three of us put our hands with fingers entwined upon his chest. Tim looked at me with so much love and softness in his eyes. He spoke of his mother, saying that he had given her the money from his brother's estate and that he had only love and compassion for her. He felt sad that she had so little experience of love in her own life.

These are the miracles that sustain us. To have been a small part of Tim's journey is to have known a hero who took on life's challenges and found the healing power of forgiveness and love. Having known the breadth and depth of Tim's raging relationship with his mother, it is a miracle that he found such peace.

PETER

I am always inspired by people's capacity to change. Change takes enormous courage. It is a step into the unknown. If one has only ever known anger as a way of dealing with life's challenges, allowing change to soften a hard and angry heart is a brave act.

Some of the more colourful characters that have come into my life have taken me all my own courage to deal with.

Not long after I first went into practice I opened my door to a man who resembled a thunderclap. It was his first appointment with me and he marched into my rooms without so much as a hello. I was suddenly very aware that I was the only person in the building at that hour. Peter carried with him a black overnight bag which he set down on the couch beside him. We went through the preliminaries of name, address, phone number, age, occupation – the usual formalities. The valuable insights that can be gleaned from these practical but seemingly inconsequential questions can be truly amazing. Insights into how we approach life can be conveyed by our body language, the way we answer a question, how much information we reveal in our answers, and so on.

Having attended to the practicalities I then said to Peter, 'Why are you here?' He responded in a way I could never have predicted. He threw the contents of the overnight bag forcibly at me. Inside there were thousands of pills of every colour – vitamins, herbs and drugs. As he threw them he screamed at me, 'I'm fucking dying and these aren't fucking helping me and now I have to come to a fuckwit woman for help!'

At that time I was very afraid of angry men because I had been hit by one. However, I knelt in front of him, put my hands on his knees and said, 'You must be very frightened.' Suddenly Peter began to sob. After a time, he told me his story.

Peter was forty-two years old; he had AIDS and no partner or friend to care for him. He felt badly done by because he had cared for others, nursing friends through their deaths; it wasn't fair that he should now be alone. Peter was an electrician by trade and he told me he had fashioned a bandanna made of foil with a timer which would end his life by electrocution at the time of his choosing.

I had recently started support and meditation groups at the Albion Street Centre in Sydney for people with HIV/AIDS and Peter began to attend. In 1985 there was enormous anger amongst gay men with HIV. This anger was largely born of fear, and their fears were more than understandable. Fear of community and family reaction; fear of the unknown; fear of disfigurement, change in body image; fear of illness, debility, suffering, dependence, rejection, abandonment, loneliness; fear of losing everyone you love. Added to all this, in some quarters, was the community attitude that they somehow deserved their unfolding horror as a punishment for who they were and the way they chose to live their lives.

Peter was really good at anger. He would express it with enthusiasm and vitality. Once, he leapt to his feet in the middle of a group and started pacing and shouting. I had to stop him by saying, 'Peter, I need you to know that I'm not with you right now because I'm afraid.'

He stopped mid-tirade. 'What are *you* afraid of?'

'I'm afraid you're going to hit me!'

'Hit you? Why would I hit you? I love you, that's why I can be angry!'

'Well, what *are* you going to hit then?'

He thought for a moment then decided, 'If I'm in the group, I'll take it out on the phone books; and if I'm in your office, I'll hit the massage table.'

Once that was clear, I felt much better, though I often used to wonder how the director of the centre felt about the volcano which would regularly erupt directly beneath his office.

For someone struggling to understand anger and to feel comfortable with her discomfort in the face of it,

Peter was a great teacher to me. He railed at the possibility of his death, judgemental community attitudes, the sensationalist media, debilitating illness and devastating loneliness.

During the eight years I knew him, Peter gradually softened. Beneath the crusty exterior, there emerged a warm, generous and loving heart. His anger gradually dissolved as he took deeper responsibility for his own perceptions of the world and began to change them. In the safe confines of the groups he expressed his anger and came to understand the fear that so often lay behind his outbursts. He was angry that there was no-one there to love and care for him, but behind his anger lay tears of loneliness and isolation. So often anger is simply a cry for help.

One image I have of him will remain with me always. Once a month, under the auspices of the Quest for Life Foundation, we organised people with life-threatening illnesses to dress up as CLOWNs – Compassion and Love Offered When Needed – and go into hospitals to entertain sick children. Peter came with us to the children's hospital and entertained a small Indonesian girl who was awaiting heart surgery. She knew no-one in Australia, except her aunt who had travelled with her. Peter was dressed as a clown with tinsel hair, sparkles in his beard, a magic wand in his hand. He could speak a little Indonesian and this frightened little girl was delighted by this colourful character who offered her words of comfort that she could understand.

In his last years Peter found a wonderful partner with whom to share his remaining life. He and Ian were regular members of our groups throughout that time. They were a loving support to one another, and gradually their love included running another support group for people with HIV who were interested in the philosophies embodied in the teachings of *A Course in Miracles*, a book which promotes a philosophical system that can help people change their perceptions.

As Peter's health deteriorated he contemplated suicide once more but dismissed it as unnecessary because he felt loved and able to surrender to the care that Ian was so keen to extend to him. He would sometimes express anger that people with AIDS have to resort to suicide. He felt that euthanasia should be available for anyone unwilling or unable to complete the last stage of their illness. His passion about taking control of his life was the impetus for these beliefs, but his outbursts became less inflamed as he focused on the precious time he and Ian had left together.

Peter's last request was that Ian care for his cat, Tiddles, in the same loving way that Peter always had. This accomplished, he rested his head on Ian's chest and surrendered his last breath, without struggle, without loneliness, without anger, without fear and with no need of the bandanna; his last words, 'I'm ready to go home now', upon his lips.

CRAIG

It may seem an obvious thing to say, but hope is healthy. Why then do so many doctors ignore this and tell patients how long they have to live? Many a person has told me that he or she has been *given* weeks or months to live. What about all the time the doctors have just *taken away* by their prognosis? Why are we so keen to ensure that people keep in the forefront of their mind the fact that they're going to die?

What is so terribly wrong with hope? Hope for a good night's rest; hope for times of laughter and love with our friends or family; hope for a remission, a cure, an afterlife?

We do not yet understand all the mechanics of how our minds interact with our bodies. At the moment what we *do* know is that we can't always change what happens to us but we certainly can play an active role in the way we respond to what happens to us.

I know hundreds of people who have far outlived their doctor's prognosis. They are spirited people who want to participate actively in their own healing process. It is time to harness the power of the mind and let it be the foundation upon which we offer choices in treatment. We need to help people find and develop their inner resources in a positive and productive way.

Surely it is better for a doctor to say: 'You have a very serious illness. Many people who have your stage of disease die within months; however, some people don't, and we want to give you all the support, treatment, skills and education so that you can be one of the ones who live long and well.'

I'd prefer that kind of doctor. She or he has simply been honest because no-one knows how long another shall live.

A supportive doctor could go further and say: 'There's much more to living well with cancer than just diagnosis and treatment. You can actively contribute to your own healing by attending a support group where you'll meet other people who've been through the experience of cancer. Look at your nutrition and make sure it's of the highest quality so that your body can cope with the treatments. It's important that you rid yourself of whatever stress you can and learn relaxation or meditation so that you manage stress as effectively as possible.'

Peace is a dynamic state in which we feel we have the best of doctors and treatments, the best support and love around us, and that there are things we can do to regain a sense of control over our lives and actively participate in our healing process. Then we can sleep with a peaceful heart, knowing that today was a day well lived and that tomorrow can be looked forward to with hope.

One Friday afternoon we were packing for one of our weekend residential programs in the country. These programs, held about eight times a year, are for people with serious illnesses and their loved ones, and are a combination of education, discussion, meditation and companionship. Usually about twenty to thirty people with cancer or other life-threatening illnesses attend, and many enduring friendships grow from these special weekends. These residential programs began in 1985 when there was a lot of community fear about AIDS and, to a lesser extent, homosexuality; in the early years about half of the participants at these programs were gay men with HIV or AIDS. However, this fact never seemed to arouse prejudices in our groups as there was a real and deep sense of camaraderie and compassion amongst those who were struggling with their own issues of mortality, suffering, meaning and purpose. One exception to this was Craig.

On this particular day we were just walking out the door when the phone rang. I decided to answer it rather than let the caller leave a message, and that is how Craig came into our lives.

He was very distressed because he'd just been told over the telephone that his melanoma had progressed rapidly and that he probably had only another six to eight weeks to live. What made this even more difficult for him was that his home, family and friends were more than a thousand kilometres away and he knew no-one in Sydney. A nurse at the hospital had given him my phone number as someone who might be able to help him.

Craig asked me bluntly over the telephone whether I could help him live because the doctors told him he was about to die.

When I told him about our weekend program and that we could organise to have someone pick him up within the hour, he jumped at the opportunity.

Craig contributed much to his first residential workshop. He began by telling the group: 'I've got a life-frightening disease. I've got a bunch of public servants for an immune system and I'm sacking the lot of them and getting in some private enterprise.' It amazed all of us that within a few short hours of being told such devastating news his humour and spirit were reasserting themselves. He was clearly in pain and the melanoma which had spread to his jaw made chewing difficult.

Craig was an opal miner and had had little experience of the city or lifestyles different from his own. He also carried with him a lot of judgement born of prejudice and fear. One of his beliefs was that 'poofters deserve to die of AIDS'.

There were three young men, Anthony, Trevor and Daniel, on the residential program who were the same age as Craig but were gay and had HIV. Craig was a little uneasy in their company; yet, in the support group, they described in their own words much of what he was feeling and hadn't as yet verbalised. They talked of their families, their loves, their hopes and disappointments, their fears and aspirations.

From this first weekend Craig made tentative friendships with these three young men who truly understood his struggles. He began to see that even though they differed from one another in disease and sexual orientation, underneath those details they faced precisely the same challenges.

Craig stayed on in Sydney for treatment and attended our support and meditation groups every week. His friendship deepened with the three boys who had initially evoked only his judgement. Craig would accompany them to their medical appointments when he could and often one or more of the boys would go with him whilst he had his radiotherapy.

Within a short time his body became so painful and difficult for him to manage that he moved into a palliative care unit near my home. Trevor, Daniel and Anthony visited him several times a week and gave him much support, encouragement and companionship. They also picked him up each week and brought him to the groups. He often used to tell me how precious it was to have them in his life because he could be real with them. They had become friends who wouldn't try to cheer him up but would let him talk about his fears and frustrations.

Once his pain was stabilised, his quality of life again improved and he was able to attend a second residential workshop in the country. His doctors continued to be pessimistic about his life expectancy. Craig would assure them that the time of his departure was strictly between himself and God and that no-one could tell him how long *they* thought *he* had to live. He'd tell them that he was already long past his use-by date or that they might know a lot about cancer but they knew precious little about *him*!

The staff at the hospice often found Craig a challenge to treat as he was impatient with his body and the limitations it created for him. His pain was as much relieved with marijuana as with morphine, but this combination was often frowned upon.

The staff were relieved when Craig's mother came from the country to be near him. Helen would spend her days at the hospice with Craig, coming home to my children and me at night because she had nowhere else to stay in Sydney. Each week Helen and Craig would attend the support and meditation groups together, Craig often lying down under a doona for the whole session as his body was too frail and painful for him to sit. Trevor, Daniel or Anthony would bring them to the groups and back again as Helen had no form of transport and needed strong physical support to manage Craig. Gradually Helen came to rely more and more on the friendship and support of her 'other boys'.

The melanoma had spread into many bones in Craig's body and several were fractured without any prospect of healing. His pelvis was already in three separate pieces and sitting or lying in one position for more than a few minutes was out of the question. Craig's determination to participate in life to the best of his ability was astounding. We knew that he would only be able to attend the group once or twice more as the ten-minute journey was becoming too much.

Imagine my surprise then when, a few weeks later, I was visiting Craig and he asked me when the next residential workshop was to be held. The next one was less than two weeks away. However, more importantly, it was held two hours from Sydney by car, with many a bump, curve and traffic jam in between. Craig had every intention of being present. He said the only reason he wouldn't be there was if he was dead. Though this was a strong possibility, I had long since given up any presumption of knowing when a person would die.

Numerous discussions followed – with his mother and sister, Donna, who had recently arrived to be with him; with the staff at the Quest for Life Centre where the groups were held, with his doctors and nursing staff, and with other members of Craig's support group.

Finally I asked Craig how he felt about a helicopter. He replied that that would be fine, just get him there. We telephoned many people in Sydney and finally it was arranged through a friend that the Australian Gas Light Company would donate the helicopter and a pilot, Laurie, for the flight to and from the workshop.

I told Laurie, 'Follow the freeway out of Mittagong and when you see the Paddy's River bridge, take a right, and a kilometre inland you'll see forty people standing in a paddock waiting for you.'

There wasn't a dry eye amongst us as we all waited for, heard and waved to the helicopter. Craig's pale face was grinning as the pilot landed the helicopter. He was gently lifted into a wheelchair which was then carried into the seminar room. Appropriately, his wheelchair was carried by his friends Trevor and Daniel whilst

Anthony held an umbrella over his head to protect him from the misty rain.

Though Craig could not participate actively in the weekend, he was the central focus for it. He was joked and smoked with, massaged and gently hugged. He mirrored powerfully to everyone present our own spirit of enthusiasm and determination. He also showed us humanity's capacity to reach beyond judgement, assumption and prejudice to find common ground where we can share the most precious parts of ourselves.

Laurie and the helicopter returned the following day to fly Craig back to the hospice. As they approached the city they saw a double rainbow over the harbour and Laurie took the helicopter up to fly right through it. Laurie didn't know that we work a lot with sending rainbows and that it had particular significance for Craig.

Craig lived another two months, mostly on the strength of telling his helicopter story. We don't judge a life by its length. It is not how long we live but the spirit with which we live that is of most importance. By this standard, Craig's short life was a triumph.

Prejudice and judgement stand in the way of us experiencing a deep and profound connection to one another. Serious illness can serve as a catalyst by which our judgements, beliefs and attitudes can be questioned and examined, then relinquished if they no longer serve us well.

BRUCE

There is little that is taboo to talk about these days. In the past, because they were rarely, if ever, discussed in public, we thought stories of child abuse must be rare, or even false. It is only now, after full and frank discussion, that we are beginning to realise the depth and extent of child abuse, and indeed other forms of physical and mental abuse perpetrated on the helpless.

People whose behaviour we deplore have, in many cases, been the victims of molesters from within their own homes or from those entrusted with their care. One such case was Bruce.

In the early years of the AIDS epidemic I worked in one of our major gaols with prisoners who were HIV positive. It was a fairly small group of men who came from different backgrounds – some were gay, some were intravenous drug users or alcoholics or both; some were first-timers but most were repeat offenders. Their crimes and sentences were also diverse – rape, murder, armed robberies, car theft, drug-trafficking and paedophilia. Their sentences ranged from three to fifteen years.

Because of their HIV status these prisoners were segregated within a maximum security gaol. Twice a week I passed through ten locked gates to reach them. Keeping them segregated was an enormous financial burden upon the system, but the mistrust and fear that most uninfected prisoners had towards them made integration a process fraught with danger.

Drugs continued to infiltrate the unit, often arriving in tennis balls hurled over the walls from within the main complex, or passed in more subtle ways. In addition, if they were on a methadone program, some of them would hide a piece of material in their mouths to soak up the drug. On returning to their cell they would remove it, squeeze it out and inject the methadone into their veins with crudely fashioned ballpoint pens.

The gaol was having difficulty in getting officers to work in the segregation unit as there was still a lot of community fear about AIDS. The tension within the unit was often more than palpable. The prospect of being sick and perhaps dying in gaol, deprived of freedom and daily contact with loved ones contributed to existing feelings of frustration and anger. Some prisoners were desperate for release to spend their remaining days with their families; some felt more secure and at home behind bars than they did outside; and others were planning the future great heist which would assure them of a comfortable end to their uncomfortable lives. The youngest was just eighteen and he'd spent the last six years in various remand centres. Needless to say, none of them seemed interested in rehabilitation or settling down to a career and a superannuation scheme on their release. There had been threats against the officers with infected blood and one successful suicide attempt amongst the prisoners.

Keeping a dozen or so men from differing backgrounds and levels of violence in a small confined space without any other contact is bound to lead to antagonisms and vented frustrations. The prisoners flushed their clothing down the toilets to block up the system in protest. The more difficult they became, the more they were locked up. The more they were locked up, the more difficult they became. Just before I was employed there were attempted suicides, bashings, arson and property damage. My job was to counsel the men with a view to calming a volatile situation and with the ultimate goal of integrating them into the main gaol.

In the early days I gained permission to take food into the prison and each week I would teach them how to cook something different. We made yoghurt and cottage cheese, bread and pumpkin pies. Trying to cut up pumpkin with a blunt plastic knife nearly drove us all to distraction until one of the prisoners removed a cupboard panel and gingerly presented me with a fairly blunt but metal kitchen knife.

While we prepared the food we would talk about anything and everything – drugs, sex, dying, living with uncertainty, relationship difficulties, grief, future plans, self-esteem and so on. It is difficult to counsel someone eye to eye when he feels intimidated by such intimate contact. It is often far easier to engage in some neutral activity so that as relaxed an environment as possible can be created. In this safe atmosphere we can begin to broach those subjects we often try to conceal. It also provides us with an opportunity to give physical expression to our feelings without involving anyone else. Sometimes I think the bread was kneaded to within an inch of its life!

Likewise, I've had some very strange conversations whilst poised to shoot pool. One of the boys, John, was particularly shy and it was a major breakthrough for him to ask me if I'd play pool with him. Just when I was about to sink a ball John asked how I'd felt when I thought I was dying. He had a close friend on the outside who was dying and John didn't know how he should be feeling.

His friend's situation was clearly a grim reminder that he too would have to face death before long. His anger and frustration at not being allowed to visit his dying friend only compounded his distorted ideas about what death might be like. I didn't sink that ball but we did sit down and have a real conversation about death and what he felt he might need to do to complete his relationship with his friend. He felt there were things he wanted to say, but he had no way of contacting him. John could neither read nor write so he hesitantly dictated a letter to me. I dared not even look at him in case it broke the spell of trust as he struggled to find the words he needed.

Once the prisoners trusted me they asked if I would facilitate a support group for them. They were very keen to have the same kind of group that I offered at the Albion Street Centre. This was somewhat of a challenge because for several weeks we had two of the prisoners segregated from the other ten because of violence between them. This meant that these two were confined to their cells whilst the others were out in the garden or recreation room, and then this was reversed. It did nothing to improve the disposition of the prisoners whose release time was curtailed because it had to be split between the two groups. It was quite impossible for me to conduct two groups as my time each week in the gaol was limited to two two-hour sessions and it was very important to make time for individual sessions too.

It might be hard to imagine but I actually conducted a support group for several weeks where ten of the prisoners were on one side of the bars and the other two on the other side. Initially the two prisoners could only listen in on the conversation, but gradually all the chairs were brought closer and closer so that, save for the bars which segregated the two prisoners, we formed a circle.

The last week before this imposed segregation was due to finish, the prisoners asked me if I was running their group in exactly the same way as the one at the Albion Street Centre. It was tremendously important to them that the services offered to people with AIDS outside the prison were replicated within the prison system. I replied that the groups were almost identical. They immediately wanted to know in what way it was different. I told them that at the beginning of the group the men at Albion Street Centre joined hands, closed their eyes and did a focusing exercise. The silence in the room was almost deafening as the boys took in this piece of information. They looked at one another and then, without a word being said, their hands came through the bars, their eyes closed and they joined together as one as I led them through a focusing exercise.

One of the prisoners was a shy, quiet man whose behaviour was exemplary and who kept very much to himself. Bruce was an avid reader and never really mixed with any of the other prisoners. He'd attend the support group but never contributed very much to the conversation. However, in our counselling time together he and I often talked about issues stimulated by the discussion in the group. He was regarded by the other prisoners with loathing because he was a rock spider, the name given to paedophiles.

The prison doctors weren't particularly concerned about Bruce's health because he had a healthy T-cell count. T-cells are the part of the immune system which is attacked by HIV. Several of the other prisoners were experiencing problems associated with HIV, but Bruce was very well. I had many conversations with him and I never found him a difficult person to like. He would occasionally talk to me about his history of paedophilia. He would describe a feeling of being taken over by this 'illness' and then he would go looking for young boys to have sex with or to molest. I was at a loss to understand his behaviour and openly shared with him my aversion to, and despair at, what he had done.

One day Bruce suddenly became ill and was diagnosed with a tumour around his spine. This lymphoma ended his life six weeks later.

Five weeks after he became ill, I made one of my regular visits to the prison. The prison officers were relieved to see me because the prisoners had been very angry and violent since they'd been released from their cells earlier in the day. They had set fire to Bruce's cell and vandalised his property and were now roaming free within the communal area.

One of the boys had punched his fist through a window which had wire embedded in the glass. His hand was covered in deep cuts and was still bleeding. Nothing frightened the officers more than the spilt blood of these prisoners, and there was no way that they would enter an area where there was blood, let alone clean it up. They were behind bars in their office and from there they had a clear view of the main recreation room but not of the cells. They assured me that if I chose to go in, they'd be watching, so long as I stayed in their view. This wasn't of enormous comfort to me.

When I entered the recreational room the boys were very upset and were pacing up and down. Their conversations were full of hatred and cruelty. They had just heard that Bruce was close to dying and they were saying how much they hoped he would have a slow and painful death. They rejoiced at his paralysis and hoped for the worst. They told me of some of the things that Bruce had done to young boys – or they thought he had done – and I felt myself becoming angry too.

Most of the boys he had molested were between ten and thirteen years of age; my own son was ten at the time. I had difficulty watching my anger and prejudices without them taking control of me. As the boys paced the floor or sat fidgeting at the table I listened to them and tried to get them to talk about their feelings. One man's anger would begin to simmer down just as another's anger would boil over. I felt I was tending a pressure cooker which could explode at any minute into terrible violence. My job was to facilitate the release of steam. Over the next two hours they gradually calmed down, stopped pacing and shouting, sat down and were finally ushered back to their cells where they were locked up. I attended to the cuts of the injured prisoner and removed all traces of his blood from his cell and the recreation room.

I continued on to the hospital to see Bruce but found that I could only spend a little time with him before I realised I would have to leave. I simply couldn't bear to be in his presence. I found feelings of loathing and disgust within myself that truly amazed me.

I went home exhausted and confused. Why was I feeling so exhausted? It was unlike me to be so tired, even after such a difficult day. I sat in my office and reflected on the feelings and events of the past few hours. I realised that the boys in gaol had only been expressing their fears. To say 'I feel afraid' is difficult because it doesn't feel strong and powerful. It also involves an awareness of our feelings and an ability to articulate them. That can be a challenge for all of us, but a willingness to be vulnerable is most certainly not a high priority for any prisoner. To hit out, to shout, to use violence, to set fire and damage property feels far more powerful than to say, 'I feel afraid because what has happened to Bruce could happen to me.'

Perhaps their thinking went something like this: 'Like me, Bruce has HIV. He has lots of T-cells. I have very few. What's to stop what's happening to Bruce, a paralysing and rapid death, from happening to me? No, it can't happen to me because I only rob banks (traffic in drugs, steal cars, rape women or whatever), I don't do dreadful things to little boys.' Having been raped myself, I know that these words will fall hard upon some women's hearts and I don't wish to intimate that rape isn't incredibly traumatic to any woman.

They had rationalised what had happened to Bruce in terms of *his* crime to reassure themselves that *their* crimes did not warrant the same physical 'punishment'; that is, a painful, paralysing death.

I also realised that when I had visited Bruce, I had been with a child molester, not with Bruce. I had brought to our meeting all my judgements, prejudices, anger and assumptions without being able to see beyond them. I chose to see something that didn't actually exist except within my own perception. And this then meant that I was relating to a person who wasn't actually there. In a way, I kept him trapped as a child molester in my interaction with him because that is whom I chose to see and relate to. Everything he said I heard through the filter of my judgement.

Bruce was sitting there as a very ill and frail man. *I* was sitting with a paedophile. I realised that I hadn't *been* with him at all, only with the illusion of who I thought he was. No wonder I was exhausted. Reality is complex and difficult enough without me adding to it!

Bruce lived another week which gave me the

opportunity of visiting him once more. When I arrived outside his hospital room I stopped, looked out the window which faced over the ocean, did some deep breathing and focused on letting go all my judgements. I sometimes do this by visualising that I'm standing inside the body of an angel or Jesus or some other being who sees the world with less judgement than I. In this case I knew I needed all the help I could get.

When I entered Bruce's room, he was sitting in a big chair, propped up with pillows. It was obvious that he was glad to see me. I pulled up a chair beside him and we settled into a companionable silence. After a time Bruce began to talk, slowly and hesitatingly at first, but with increasing energy and enthusiasm. We talked for two hours.

During that time he told me the story of his life. He told it in a way I had never heard it before. He talked of his childhood where he was brutally abused, molested and raped. He had lived with his father who was an alcoholic and who regularly sexually abused him. In addition several of his father's friends regularly had 'sessions' with Bruce in which he was molested, raped and brutally beaten. Bruce told me about hiding in the gardening shed or the outhouse amongst spiders and other fearful things of the dark. But none of them was nearly as bad as being found by his father or one of his friends.

How can we know the extent of another's pain or how that pain will affect their subsequent actions? Bruce told me how throughout his life, this 'illness' would come over him and he would feel compelled to molest young boys.

Several times, when he stopped to rest and draw breath, he'd say to me, 'I've never told anyone any of this before. Is it alright for me to keep talking?' I assured him it was and that I wanted to hear more.

Bruce talked about the whole history of his life and finally came to the present moment, to his being in prison, ill and dying. He then looked very directly into my eyes and completely rocked me by saying, 'I've become a Christian and I've asked for forgiveness for what I've done to young boys and I *have* accepted it.'

I was stunned, and inside myself a voice said, 'How dare you accept forgiveness for what you have done?' I was amazed to find a part of myself that wanted Bruce to suffer forever.

I refrained from uttering the words of my judgement and brought myself back into the present moment. I looked at him with humility, awe and gratitude. Surely the anger and judgement I could have so easily turned upon Bruce was no more nor less than the judgements I held against myself. Of course I was horrified by his actions, but Bruce taught me the extent of my own self-judgement. In fact, without Bruce, I cannot fathom or get in touch with the amount of self-judgement I hold onto; to find the part of myself which feels unforgivable, that feels that it doesn't deserve to exist or, conversely, that believes I'm somehow better than other people. Our judgement of others only serves to maintain the belief that we are separate from one another. When we let go our judgement we can experience a deep sense of connection which allows our compassionate nature to flow more easily. In this way it becomes easy to love the being that has made a difficult journey, whilst not necessarily liking the actions of that being.

I hugged Bruce gently, thanked him for sharing his story and bade him farewell. I felt privileged to have had the opportunity of knowing him. He died very peacefully a short while after our conversation.

To say, 'I have asked for forgiveness, and I have accepted it,' and to have that deeply heard by another person, without judgement, must surely be extraordinary when all you have ever experienced is other people's anger and derision. Perhaps the opportunity Bruce had to speak of his life, knowing that there was no judgement, somehow completed his healing and released the pain of his past.

For some people, this story will be beyond comprehension or acceptance. I am in no way implying that Bruce's actions were forgivable or acceptable. Bruce was a child molester and needed to be kept away from people he might harm; being in gaol was exactly the right place for him to be, dying under guard was appropriate. To forgive the person does not mean to forgive his actions. With understanding and compassion it is possible to see beyond the behaviour to the wounded being within. Surely to create a safe environment in which that wounded being can begin to heal is to create the possibility of a better future for us all.

I know that when I'm able to leave judgement at the door, strange and unexpected things happen. I also know this brings comfort to both me and the person I am listening to, and often a new perception of life as well. It's the essence of forgiveness to leave judgement aside and see the person or situation afresh, letting go of perceptions, and expectations and simply allowing oneself to be present to them.

TAMARA

The phone rang and the conversation went like this.

'Hello, I'm Tamara and I can't keep anything down. Can you help?'

'Perhaps, Tamara. Would you like to come and see me?'

'Yes, but I can't walk.'

'Would you like me to come and see you at home?'

'Yes, please.'

'Tamara, is there a reason why you can't keep anything down or why you can't walk?'

'Oh yes, I've had cancer.'

Tamara's husband met me at the door. The smell of fresh-brewed coffee followed us up steep steps to an upper storey and into a beautiful sunny room overlooking a tree-filled garden.

Propped up in bed amongst a mountain of pillows

was a woman in her early forties. Her fingernails were bright red talons and she had a diamond studded cigarette holder elegantly poised between her fingers in preparation for her next draw. Diamonds hung from her ear lobes and her lips matched the colour of her fingernails. Tamara had soulful eyes that were fully made up and she peered out under false eyelashes. Her hair was carefully arranged and held in place by a beautiful comb and spray. She smelt of Chanel No 5, though I detected a whiff of something else which clearly had not come out of a French perfume bottle. When I looked a little closer it was obvious that Tamara's hair and make-up had been applied with great care but by shaky fingers and that her nail polish covered more than her fingernails alone. Beside her bed was a glass of coke and a strategically placed bowl covered by an embroidered cloth. It was obvious to me that Tamara was very close to dying.

Joe was a loving partner doing his best to take care of someone he clearly adored. He'd organised to have indefinite leave from his company so that he could care for Tamara, and out of his own desperation and worry he chose to believe every word she said. She told him that she was getting better and that she'd be fine, and he believed her absolutely. Joe's days were filled with cooking, cleaning and caring for Tamara, and he said he was happy to be allowed to be this close to her – a comment I found strange at the time and would only understand later.

Tamara had told him only the parts of her medical history that she had chosen to hear. She had heard her doctors say things like 'We have removed most of the tumour in your abdomen' and 'You have responded very well to your treatment' and 'The radiotherapy has been very effective'. What she hadn't heard was that they had not been able to remove all the tumour from her uterus and that, though she had responded well to her treatment, the doctors never expected to cure her of her disease. She was most certainly beyond the hope of chemotherapy or radiotherapy.

These two people were remarkably isolated from the community because of their love of privacy, and I realised that no-one was involved in Tamara's medical care any more. The surgeon had completed his job and had passed her along to the chemotherapist for further treatment. On completion of that she had been referred to a radiation oncologist, and at the end of her two-week radiation therapy she was on her own.

In addition Joe and Tamara had distanced themselves from friends because they had wanted time to devote themselves to Tamara's recovery and to be alone together. Joe would speak to friends who dropped in either at the front door or occasionally invite them into the kitchen for coffee, but no-one but Joe had ascended the stairs to Tamara's bedroom in weeks. Joe would deliver the flowers, messages or love from those who called, but he had adhered to Tamara's wishes that no-one should see her until she was 'on top of things'.

Undoubtedly, after she had completed her treatment she had been referred back to her GP or to another oncologist, but Tamara, believing that she had pursued all her treatment options, carried on with her life as if cancer were a thing of the past. She had found her treatments a challenge as how she looked was of tremendous importance to her. Joe adored her no matter how she looked, but Tamara desperately needed to appear elegantly dressed and presentable at all times. It was unthinkable to appear dishevelled. The moment she woke up, she got up to attend to her face and hair. That was now almost impossible, although Joe would bring her a bowl of warm water and her make-up bags so that she could attend to those details in privacy.

Joe was finding it a struggle to help Tamara down the three steep steps that led to their ensuite. When I witnessed one of these journeys to the bathroom I was amazed that they both hadn't suffered injuries! Tamara's balance was gone and she barely had the strength to lift a foot; in fact, Joe lifted each foot for her as they went.

In Tamara's mind her needs were simple. She wanted to get the nausea under control, then she'd be able to eat and she would get her strength back; if she had her strength, her walking would be fine, and she and Joe could continue their loving relationship. There was no crack in the armour of her beliefs and to talk of her impending death would have been cruel and unnecessary.

Under stress, people generally conduct themselves in the very best way they know how. Given the strains that a life-threatening illness places upon those involved, it is not surprising that our defences are at their strongest and most effective. I have never felt it my place to break down people's defences. They are clearly in place for a very good reason. I prefer to help create a truly safe environment, free of judgement or any agenda, so that a person might feel safe enough to explore their own issues and let go their defences when they see no further need for them.

I was very mindful of establishing a trusting relationship with Tamara in order for us to be able to give her the more intensive care that I knew she would very shortly need. It was obvious that the only person she trusted was Joe, but she was also aware that she needed some practical help which Joe simply could not offer. She was reluctant to tell me any details of her medical history, believing it to be a thing of the past, and the only hint she gave me was the information that she had had surgery and radiotherapy to her abdomen and that she now had a discharge from her vagina. I could only imagine how distressing she would find anything which might compromise her dignity and femininity. It was Joe who told me that her cancer had first been detected in her uterus.

We talked about some dietary guidelines which would help decrease her nausea, though I knew she was really beyond eating. I suggested flat lemonade rather than coke. I didn't mention her smoking as it was clear that her ability to continue doing so would shortly cease.

Tamara had had a falling out with her GP over something she couldn't remember. I thought it most likely that the GP had said things Tamara simply didn't want to hear. She would not let me contact her GP and wanted nothing further to do with her. She hadn't seen any doctor for more than three months and relied on Joe's pain medication prescribed for his back to ease the minimal pain and discomfort she experienced. Contrary to many people's beliefs, cancer does not always produce pain. Tamara's discomfort was more from the stiffness of her joints as she lay mostly immobile in her bed.

I eased into the subject of getting medical help by suggesting that there was some equipment which could make bathing and toileting far simpler. Tamara didn't like the sound of a commode chair at all and recoiled at the idea of having 'a toilet in the bedroom'. She said that getting to the bathroom wasn't a problem! I could see that they were very hesitant about having anyone else in their home.

Tamara's answers to my questions were abrupt, which made it very difficult to turn anything into a conversation, let alone a discussion. As a way of creating a space in which she might talk a little more about her present state, her life or her illness, I suggested that I could give her a massage. Her reaction amazed me.

In a most indignant voice she replied, 'No, thank you!'

I looked at Joe who gave me a knowing look and said, 'She hates to be touched. I can hardly ever get close to her.'

Not persuaded, I asked her, 'Have you ever had a massage?'

'No,' she replied.

'Well, why don't I massage just one foot and if you don't like it, I won't do the other one?'

I had chosen the foot because it somehow seemed less threatening. Tamara reluctantly agreed and Joe left us alone whilst I massaged cream into her foot. Needless to say, one foot and she was a goner for massage! She happily surrendered the other foot to my care.

We sat in silence during the massage and I made sure my movements were slow, firm and comforting. Whenever I massage anyone's feet I feel a sense of reverence for these often overlooked parts of our bodies and for the journey they have helped us to make.

I had noticed when I entered Tamara's bedroom that on Joe's bedside table there was a copy of my book, *Quest for Life*. After several minutes of silence, whilst I massaged her second foot, Tamara said, 'What was it like when you thought you were dying?' At last.

I replied that I'd found it a scary experience because it was full of the unknown, but I was grateful because it had taught me a lot about life and what was really important.

Tamara seemed satisfied with my response and settled back to doze whilst I finished her massage. When I straightened the bedclothes and prepared to leave, Tamara was instantly awake and asked if I would return the following day. I agreed to return in the morning and told her she could call me any time if she needed to reach me before then.

I headed downstairs to Joe, hoping to have a conversation with him about his and Tamara's needs. He was more open to having help because he wanted the best for her and could see that his resources were wearing thin.

When I told him of Tamara's question during our massage he said that, as far as he knew, that was the only conversation Tamara had ever had about dying. She certainly had never mentioned it as a possibility to him.

He then asked me bluntly whether she was dying. I replied that she was, as he knew, very ill, and that perhaps she might only have a short time to live. It is hard to see someone completely crumple and Joe seemed suddenly to age ten years. I hastened to add that I was unqualified to make any pronouncements and that I felt the need for medical support to ensure that Tamara would be as comfortable as possible.

Joe immediately responded with absolute certainty that he wanted to take care of Tamara himself. I asked him to think about our conversation and to let me know the following morning what he had decided. I also suggested that it was important to make contact with anyone Tamara might want to see before she died. He mumbled something about an estranged relationship with her father, who was her only living relative. Joe had never met him and he had no idea why Tamara had become estranged from him. There had been no argument, no crisis, just a drifting away from each other. Joe was clearly anxious to return to Tamara's bedside so I left.

On my arrival the following morning I spoke with Joe before we went upstairs. Tamara had slept quite well even though it was necessary for Joe to change the bed twice because of soiling. Nothing seemed to faze him and the way he tended to her unpleasant discharge was as if he were dealing with the nectar of the gods. I had brought with me some pads that would be more effective and some other bits and pieces that I knew we would either need or would make caring for Tamara easier.

I asked Joe if he had thought about our conversation and if he was willing to have the palliative care team involved in Tamara's care. He said that he would rely on me to provide the minimal amount of medical support they might need. He wanted no strangers involved but would be willing to have any equipment which could be helpful in caring for Tamara. I assured him that I felt I needed the support of the nurses and he was willing, in fact grateful, to surrender to my better judgement.

I was concerned that if we became bogged down in Tamara's medical management we might lose the opportunity to create the peaceful environment she and Joe really wanted. For instance, had a doctor been called, she might have insisted that Tamara's discharge be dealt with differently, but it was important to Joe to offer Tamara the kind of care she could accept. There's much more to dying than the medical perspective. Had she been in pain, in need of oxygen or any other medical assistance, I would have been the first to have recommended such intervention.

It was clear to me that Tamara and Joe weren't at all interested in a medical perspective, so my aim became to assist them complete whatever they needed to with dignity and with as little emotional and physical suffering as possible.

I had spoken to the nurses and explained the complexities of Joe and Tamara's ways of dealing with things. The palliative care nurses are used to dealing with complicated or idiosyncratic relationships and agreed to come to their home, review Tamara's medical needs, provide what equipment might be necessary, then remain in the background for assistance if that was required.

As soon as I entered Tamara's room she greeted me like a long-lost friend and said she was ready for her massage. I began with her feet and then suggested that her neck and shoulders looked a little cramped and perhaps she would let me give them a bit of a rub. She was ready to take whatever I had the time to give. Two hours later she looked like she was in heaven.

The palliative care nurses arrived and briefly met Tamara, although she wouldn't allow them to examine her. They left some equipment, including the dreaded commode, and the next time Tamara needed the toilet she was grateful for its proximity.

Her deterioration was now very rapid and I was concerned that Joe felt out of his depth with the responsibility of Tamara's care. He told me he had contacted her father against her wishes because he felt her death would come as a terrible shock if he were not informed until after the event. Her father was due to arrive from interstate at eleven the following morning. When I offered to sleep over and be on hand should he need me, my offer was leapt upon by both him and Tamara.

We changed Tamara's pads many times throughout the night as the discharge increased dramatically. We were able to do this with minimal disturbance to Tamara and Joe's un-wavering tender care of her was quite outstanding. As dawn crept closer Tamara drifted beyond words and her breathing became irregular. We washed her gently and attended to her needs.

Her eyes were closed and I wondered, as we lavished

attention on her body, where she might be. I massaged her feet, her hands, her back and neck, and then settled beside her to watch and wait. Joe was still struggling with the finality of these hours and resorted to fidgeting, pacing, smoking and making endless cups of coffee. I silently mused on the similarities between birth and death and how the labour that produces either result is hard on those who are relegated to the place of witness. I encouraged him to say to Tamara whatever was in his heart, but all he could do was weep.

One of the ways that I find very helpful in joining with someone who is beyond words is to take on their breathing pattern. It helps to enter into their 'time zone' and I did with this Tamara. After a short time, and while Joe was out of the room, I said to her, 'You might see a beautiful light.' Her eyes immediately flew open and went to the window where the morning sun was just establishing itself. Then her gaze fastened on my eyes and twinkled with enormous presence and peace. I welcomed her back and reassured her that all was well and that she was doing fine. She twinkled in reply.

Joe returned to the bedroom and seemed much comforted by the fact that Tamara's eyes were open and focused. It was as if he felt his connection with her was re-established. He told her that her father was coming at eleven and it was obvious that, though she could not respond, she understood precisely what he had said. There was a momentary hesitation to the twinkle in her eyes and then it returned as Joe took my place on the floor beside the bed, held onto her hand and began to talk to her hesitatingly.

On the one hand I knew my presence gave great reassurance to Joe and possibly even to Tamara, although perhaps she was beyond needing me. However, the moments around a person's death can be incredibly precious as things are said and done that are full of the intimacy of a loving relationship. To have so recently entered into these people's lives and now to be involved in such shared intimacy was a humbling privilege.

As Joe began to whisper to Tamara I endeavoured to make my presence as invisible as possible. He said to her, and I know he won't mind me sharing this with you: 'Sweet darling, take from all the love that surrounds you right now and do with it whatever you need to. If you need to leave, it's alright for you to go. If you want to stay, I'll be here for you. I'll be OK, you'll be OK, and we'll meet again.' My heart felt full and ready to break at the sound of his words and the love they conveyed.

I continued with my practice of breathing in rhythm with Tamara and during the morning she stopped breathing three times. Each time she stopped I reassured her that she was doing fine and that she could simply relax and let go; she didn't need to hang onto anything. The joy that emanated from her eyes was indescribable. Each time her sparkling eyes stayed focused on mine or on Joe's and her breathing would start up again. I have rarely experienced such awareness and presence in someone so close to death. I marvelled at the inner journey Tamara had made in the space of less than forty-eight hours and I gave thanks for the privilege of this work.

At eleven Tamara's father arrived to bid his farewell and Tamara sparkled in response. Before her father had left the room, Tamara had left her body. Even at the very end of life, acknowledging one another in peace and acceptance can transform the history of a relationship.

We must be careful of the presumptions we make about another's journey and the choices they make as they struggle with illness and the finality of death. Tamara could easily have been classified as being in denial, and yet she conducted herself through her debilitating illness with her dignity and self-respect intact. To this day, hers was one of the most aware and conscious departures of any person I've worked with.

So often we want to make life neat and tidy in the hope that it gives us control of what happens to us. If we can explain away an illness or tragedy, then we might believe we're in a position to understand the ways in which we can prevent the same tragedy or illness from happening to us. That's why my favourite bumper sticker is *My karma just ran over your dogma.*

Life isn't neat and tidy, and people behave in the manner which is consistent with who they are. If we can respectfully enter into another's inner life, we can catch a glimpse of the world through their eyes. Perhaps then we can offer a word of comfort or through a gesture convey the respect and honour that every person deserves.

In order to offer compassionate care to another human being we must take the time to know and understand them and not try to bend them to our wishes. To presume to know what is best for another, without a clear understanding of who they are, is to miss the opportunity for learning and being an integral part of their intimate journey into the mystery of death.

ROMA AND DENNIS

Roma and Dennis were best friends. I find it impossible to think of Roma without thinking of Dennis. These two were peas in a pod. They belonged to one another in a rare and precious way. Their relationship was one which I admired enormously. Their marriage was based upon a deep and abiding friendship.

The two met in 1949 in Roma's brother Sonny's shop where she and her sister Nella were working together. Dennis asked her out twice. Roma flatly refused. Dennis gave it one last shot and she succumbed. They married two years later and became virtually inseparable from then on.

In 1983, out of the blue, Roma felt a pain in her abdomen. At first the doctors thought she had appendicitis, however, it turned out to be cancer of the colon. The surgeon was confident that the cancer had been completely removed and Roma and Dennis resumed their happy lives together. Seven years later Roma developed a dry cough whilst holidaying in Italy, Roma's homeland. On their return to Australia Dennis insisted that she consult a doctor about her cough. The doctors suspected tuberculosis. The couple were devastated to find that Roma's cancer had returned and that during surgery to the lung the surgeon had found other tumours which he could not remove.

Their GP recommended meditation, and Roma and Dennis came into my life. We liked one another immediately. Roma had an extraordinary capacity to love people and to make each person feel important. She was a people person. She never asked for sympathy, never complained and always had a whimsical way about her. Often she would say, 'I'll be better tomorrow.' She didn't say that to cheer up others, it was a belief she had complete faith in.

For more than five years Roma shared her philosophy, humour, vulnerability, insights, tears and wisdom with the meditation group she attended weekly in my home. There were up to fifty people with life-threatening illnesses who would attend this group each week. The room comfortably held about thirty people and when the group exceeded that number it was filled wall to wall, with people under the tables, on cushions, in chairs, on sofas and stretched out on the floor. The sense of camaraderie was something to behold. Someone who was unwell would happily give up their chair or cushion to someone sicker than they. Together we grieved for many of the participants who attended the group, knowing that each time we mourned the loss of one of our members, it was a grim reminder of our own fragile hold on life.

Roma and Dennis gradually came to be like the mum and dad of the group, always arriving early and making sure that everyone was comfortable, fetching glasses of water or cushions for those who needed them, and warmly welcoming newcomers and getting them settled. Roma amazed me with her ability to be wholeheartedly present and attentive when someone was sharing their story, regardless of her own discomfort. She was not only attentive, but could always offer some words of encouragement or understanding. Everyone in the groups loved Roma and Dennis, their sense of humour and the warmth and love they showed to one another and to each person as they arrived.

Finally Roma could no longer attend the groups as she was too breathless and weak to make the journey from her home to mine. At the conclusion of the meditation practice each week the group would send Roma and Dennis a rainbow. This practice might sound a little strange to some, but we always draw strength from it and it helps us to maintain a sense of connection and support, enabling us to extend our love and blessings across the rainbow.

I started visiting Roma on a regular basis, and this became more frequent as her health continued to deteriorate. Dennis insisted on taking care of all Roma's physical needs and did so with great tenderness. He had promised to keep her at home and through his loving care she remained in her own beloved house and garden.

No-one could care for another any better than Dennis did. The love and devotion that flowed effortlessly between the two of them was a joy to be around.

Every morning Roma would stand on their balcony overlooking the bushland that surrounded their home and greet the day. She would say, 'Good morning, morning' and look forward to another day with Dennis. She would talk to the lorikeets and her plants and always encourage them. In all the years I knew Roma I never heard her speak ill of anyone and she had a marvellous capacity to see the good or positive in any situation. You simply could nor resist loving her because she made you feel so good. She was enormously loved by many people and, of course, especially so by Dennis.

Roma and I had many discussions about death, dying, what lies beyond death and the awful impending separation from Dennis that loomed on a distant but ever-closer horizon. Her Catholic beliefs gave her a faith but it didn't extend to any regular attendance at church.

Some days she couldn't believe that she and Dennis could ever part; other days, when each breath was difficult, she ached for release from a body which no longer functioned without struggle and assistance. She worried over Dennis's ability to cook and would sit at the table giving him step-by-step guidance in food preparation. He never took her seriously because he never really thought she'd die. So long as she was alive, he would take care of her.

Even though, towards the end of her life, much of her time was spent in bed, it was more usual to hear laughter than sadness when you entered her bedroom.

Every visit I had with her, she would always find something to laugh about. There were plenty of sad times too, but Roma never let you leave her feeling down or disheartened.

The last time I spoke to Roma her concerns were not about her own suffering but about the loss she knew Dennis would feel at their parting. It was typical of her to be preoccupied by thoughts of someone else. She would say to him, 'I feel I want to go for a long sleep.' He knew what she meant but he would reply, 'Just have a little doze.'

She loved her bubble baths and her porridge. On her last day Dennis carried her to her bath, cooked her porridge and then, at her request, asked Dennis to call her family together so she could say her goodbyes.

Roma died peacefully that evening and Dennis telephoned to let me know. I offered to come over to their home immediately, but Dennis said that he wanted the evening to themselves and to sleep beside his love one more time. Something in the way Dennis expressed this wish alerted me to the difficulty he might have in letting go of Roma. I suggested a couple of practical things for Dennis to do so that the bedding would be protected, and we agreed that I'd come early the following morning. I was keen to see Dennis as I knew how incomprehensible Roma's death would be for him. There were also practical details to be arranged as Roma had asked me some months before if I would conduct her funeral.

When I arrived, Dennis and I hugged and he took me in to see Roma. The room was very still and Dennis had lit a candle amongst some of Roma's treasures on the dressing table. She looked very much at peace and quite beautiful; the lines of struggle on her face had melted and her skin had taken on a translucent glow.

Dennis spoke lovingly to Roma as if she was able to hear, though, I noticed, he didn't expect any response. He said that she looked as if she were just dozing, and the loving softness in his eyes gave no indication of the reality of their parting. Again I felt some concerns about Dennis's ability to separate and let Roma go.

Like most people, Dennis was fairly uninformed about what needs to happen when someone dies, but he had some strong ideas about who should care for Roma's body and how.

Sometimes doing something practical together can help us to take on board the physical fact of death, so I suggested to Dennis that we wash Roma's body together. He was keen to continue caring for her and this idea appealed to him.

We tended her body with gentleness and respect and I was grateful that we were able to perform this last gesture for our friend together. Dennis too was thankful that we had each other and we talked quietly whilst we attended to the task at hand. He would often stop as we worked and look at her as if his heart would melt with loving tenderness. We dressed her in a beautiful suit she had not long ago worn to a wedding and, with encouragement from Dennis, I made up her face in the manner she liked.

Dennis spoke in his usual warm and loving way and didn't seem at all thunderstruck by Roma's death. He still says that even now he hasn't come to terms with her death and that he never believed that she wouldn't recover. No matter how much we prepare ourselves for the death of a loved one, it always comes as a shock when that person finally dies. Even if we have years of preparation, when death finally comes, so does the tremendous shock of disbelief. It's as if we can't actually prepare for the fact of death, even if it has been long predicted.

Dennis and I sat at the dining room table to discuss the details of Roma's funeral. I encouraged him to have things the way he would like them, whilst taking into account Roma's expressed wishes.

By the time I left I felt more confidence in Dennis's ability to let Roma go, though he had often reverted to speaking of her as if she were still alive and only sleeping.

I wanted to stay until Roma's body was taken from the house but I had to leave because I had a support group to facilitate. I promised to return that afternoon to finalise the details of Roma's cremation.

Dennis called the funeral home and told them that he had lost his beloved wife. They replied by asking him when he wanted them to pick up the body. Dennis felt outraged and told them this was not about a body, it was about his wife.

Dennis wanted Roma placed directly into the coffin in which she was to be cremated. Usually the undertakers remove the body in a temporary coffin, or a body bag, attend to the body, and place it in the chosen coffin at the funeral home. Dennis told them that they didn't need to do anything to her as we had attended to all her needs and that he wanted them to bring the coffin to the house so that he could see her safely ensconced, knowing that she need not be disturbed again.

Dennis also wanted the funeral cars to deviate from their usual route to the crematorium so that they could pass by their home for one last time. He wanted to walk with the undertaker in front of the funeral car as it passed their house.

Dennis asked for the cross that adorned Roma's coffin to be mounted as a keepsake. He asked for the north chapel of the crematorium because their home faced north, and the niche he chose for her final resting place also faced the same direction. Dennis had Roma's funeral service printed into a beautiful booklet with her photograph at the front so that those who remembered her with love would have something of her to keep. All these things Dennis did. Each of them was important in coming to terms with the finality of his parting from Roma.

Dennis and I have remained friends and I'm sure we always will. There's much talk about remaining emotionally detached from the people we work with professionally. I believe this is both unrealistic and unnecessary. We constantly react to one another, and by sharing our stories and our journeys we learn more from one another than we would if we remained aloof and emotionally uninvolved. Through this deeper sharing of ourselves we discover ways to live through crisis, change, loss, trauma, grief and sadness. In fact, I believe that burnout is the end result of stifling our emotions. We all need to find a safe harbour in which we can express how we feel. Any health professional fulfilling the role of counsellor also needs to find a safe harbour in which to replenish and centre themselves.

As Dennis found, we need rituals as ways of celebrating life's momentous occasions. Through rituals we gradually release the pain of our parting and, though our loved one is never forgotten, we are more able to greet the day and participate in it.

TONY

Not all abuse is physical or sexual. Mental abuse can be every bit as damaging and difficult to recover from. Often recovery is a lifelong task.

In 1984 I started a voluntary massage program for people with AIDS at one of Sydney's major hospitals. It had struck me that to be very ill and, in addition, to feel that no-one wanted to touch me, would be unbearable. Tony was the first person I massaged and he was seventeen years old. Throughout the massage he wept silently, the puddle on his pillow gradually increasing until I began to wonder whether the massage was a mistake.

When I'd finished I asked him if he wanted to talk about his tears. His reply saddened and shocked me. 'No-one has ever touched me like that before. I've only ever been touched when someone wanted something from me.'

His story tumbled out. He'd been thrown out of home at fifteen because he was gay; he hated his parents and had no intention of telling them where he was or that he was very ill. He was full of bitterness and resentment about his life, his family, HIV and his sexuality.

After his release from hospital Tony came regularly to our support and meditation groups where he dealt with his anger at himself, his life and his family. At first he found the group quite confronting as many of the participants were thin and frail. He rang me to talk about this discomfort with people who were clearly sicker than he. Yet there was nowhere else he could go and be listened to about the issues he wished to explore. Tony assured me that he would never allow himself to go through the thin and frail part of his illness and drew comfort from the fact that he had the knowledge of how to take his own life when he thought the time was right. This reassured him sufficiently to overcome his fear of participating in the group.

I wasn't particularly alarmed at Tony's words as many of the participants felt the same way. Suicide and euthanasia were spoken of almost on a weekly basis in the AIDS group. I felt that it was imperative that the group members had a safe environment in which they could discuss their fears, concerns and plans for the future, for where else were they to talk? It is difficult for many people to understand what it felt like for these young men who lived in a world in which most of their friends, partners, acquaintances and lovers were sick, dead, dying or living with HIV. Some had lost everyone they called a friend and they had little reason to feel passionate about living.

Many a participant had uttered the same words as Tony about ending their own life before they became their own worst nightmare. But they continued to come to the groups for years. As time passed, they adjusted to their many physical losses and, years down the track, they'd be sitting in the group, thin and frail, but content with their quality of life.

At seventeen Tony was still coming to terms with his sexuality; his feelings compounded by the disease which his few experiments with sex had given him. Tony railed at his sexual confusion and the fact that AIDS would now rob him of both his ability to have children and, indeed, his life. Like many, he found that behind his anger were tears of the hurt and pain of his family's judgement of him and sadness about the mess he felt his life was in. Tony's life had only just begun and yet he now had to face his mortality. He kept a journal of his feelings and, through his writing, gradually let go of his anger and bitterness. With the impetus of his declining health and many tears, he released his shame, gradually reclaiming his dignity and finding the ability to extend forgiveness to himself and others. He wrote letters to his family in which he expressed his feelings, extended his forgiveness to them and asked for their acceptance of him. It was amazing to witness the peace which seemed to have settled in his heart and the sparkle which now danced in his eyes.

Years later Tony called me and asked me to come and say goodbye. I walked into the very same room as I had four years previously and there, massaging his feet, was his mother; his father, lost in his own thoughts as his son rested, sat stroking Tony's hand, and his sister was by his side reading. The love and harmony in the room was palpable.

I went to his side and he immediately awoke. I gently massaged his belly for a while as it was terribly distended. He finally removed his oxygen mask and beckoned me close as he could to whisper: 'It's been wonderful knowing you. Thank you for teaching me about love. These have been the best four years of my life.'

It is easy to say it's a tragedy when a person dies at such a young age. Yet, to live for ninety years with a lifetime of bitterness, fear, resentment and unresolved issues is a far greater tragedy. Had he lived so long, Tony may never have found his peace. His parents could have died with their relationship with their son unresolved. Through AIDS, Tony and his family found one another again. No-one could not be deeply moved and saddened by his life; but out of it came love, healing, peace and ultimately reconciliation. I believe that Tony died healed of everything that ever stood in the way of his peace. Paradoxically, it was AIDS that was the catalyst for that deeper healing.

ANGUS

People can give away an extraordinary amount of information about themselves without so much as uttering a word. Volumes can be conveyed through posture, the way we enter a room, the chair we choose to sit in, our clothing and personal appearance, the spring in our step or the lack of it, the lines on our face or the state of our hands.

On his first visit Angus sat very stiffly in my waiting room with a briefcase on his knee and glasses perched upon the end of his nose. He wore a suit and tie, polished shoes and had beautifully manicured fingers and hands, which showed he never did any manual work. His wife, Gillian, sat on another couch in the waiting room and it wasn't at first evident that they were together, let alone married. He stood up abruptly when I spoke his name and followed me into my room without a backward glance at his wife. Gillian looked harassed and distracted and followed Angus and me with all the enthusiasm of someone on their last day on death row.

When Angus first entered my office I felt he had come to interrogate me and that he wanted to take charge of our time together. I almost felt as though I should offer him my chair and desk and that I should sit elsewhere.

I always sit facing the person with whom I am conversing, but Angus moved his chair slightly before he sat down so that my desk was between us. He neatly arranged his briefcase on his knees, flicked open the catches and took out a notepad with a list of numbered questions. He carefully closed the briefcase, straightened all the edges of the notepad, took out a pen and peered at me over his glasses. Gillian pretended not to exist as she quietly mangled the strap of her handbag.

Angus launched into his story with precision and gusto. He had recently had to give up his position as a lecturer in statistical analysis because he had been diagnosed with cancer of the oesophagus. He had undergone extensive surgery and was quite debilitated. He was seeking guidance from me as to his nutrition and wanted to know if he was meditating correctly.

As he told me his story it was as if he was speaking of someone else. The details were conveyed in a matter-of-fact tone and it was clear that he was only interested in giving me his clinical summations rather than giving out any information about his feelings. Angus told me that he intended to return to work as soon as possible even though he had actually taken early retirement from the university because of his health.

There was so much controlled anger and frustration in him that it seemed quite pointless to discuss anything before addressing his immediate state. I wondered whether Angus would let me in at all to the turbulent world he so clearly lived in. I glanced at Gillian whose eyes shifted nervously and then dropped to the floor.

Where to begin? I decided to ask him about his work, knowing that he would feel quite safe with this familiar territory. Gradually we moved on to talking about his farewell from the university, and when I enquired about the reception held for him and what they had said to him at his departure, his face softened just a little and he almost smiled. They had been very appreciative of his years of service and some of his students had written him letters which had quite moved him. I remarked that he was obviously passionate about his subject and he launched into a description of what was involved in statistical analysis. Gillian concentrated on the shredding of her handbag strap as Angus warmed to his subject.

Obviously he and Gillian had been thrown together in a far more intense way than they had ever experienced before. When he drew breath, I turned to Gillian and asked her how it was to have Angus at home all the time. She looked as if someone might strike her and before she could utter a word, Angus literally spat out the words, 'She's trying to kill me!'

'How so?' I asked.

Angus felt that if only his wife would do things the way he liked them to be done, or in the way he would do them – implying, of course, that this would be the right way – he would be able to get well. In his view, she was killing him by her non-cooperation. This extended from how she washed the dishes, to how she answered the phone, to keeping the kids quiet whilst he furiously meditated! He had conducted time and motion studies of most of her activities at home and poor Gillian had come up very short.

I returned my attention to Gillian, who could only mutter that she found it a great strain to have him at home all day watching how she did things.

If any healing was to take place in this man, it was clear it must begin within the family and his own attitudes before it would even be worthwhile contemplating changes to his diet. To talk about vegetable juice at a time when serious injury might be inflicted by the juicer in flight would be totally inappropriate. Furthermore, he could hardly drink juice through his clenched teeth.

As we continued to talk it became obvious, even to Angus, that because he had little control over what was happening in his body, he was fighting hard to exert control over something else. Gillian and the way she ran the home had become his target and he relentlessly pursued his new career of home manager. Being a statistician didn't help. Numbers move along very prescribed lines. In his mind Angus had decided that if he couldn't control what was happening in his body, then he would control – to within an inch of his life – what was happening in his external environment.

People may use blame for many different reasons but

each and every one will come back to not wanting to own their responsibility. Society reinforces this attitude in many ways. We blame the weather. We blame circumstances. We blame other people. We blame society. We go out of our way to avoid taking responsibility. When we accept our responsibility it means we decide to make changes in our lives. If we continue to blame outside circumstances, what we are really saying is, 'If only *you* would change, I would be happier.'

During our sessions together over the following months Angus's attitude softened and he began to talk a lot more about his father and their relationship. His father, who had been a bricklayer all his life, had been a very demanding person who had insisted on a 'do it once and do it well' approach to everything.

Even on their fishing trips together Angus's father always corrected him on how he tied his hook to the line or how he made a fly for fishing trout. He would check everything Angus did and would never let an opportunity pass if he could pass on his 'wisdom' or give his son guidance on the proper way to do things. Angus admitted that he was quite frightened of him and that his relationship with his father now was nonexistent. When his father would drink too much he would be bad-tempered and tell Angus that he would never amount to anything. Angus hadn't seen him for several years and his father, who now suffered with Alzheimer's disease, lived interstate in a nursing home.

In time Angus was also able to acknowledge that it was his father who had pushed him into his studies and, finally, into a career which had given him both acclamation and satisfaction.

Angus's relationship with his own son, Michael, was strained and, though he'd sworn he would never be like his own father, Angus gradually realised that he too placed many conditions on his love for Michael. He would focus on the marks that were lost in Michael's school studies rather than on the marks won. Michael's athletic achievements were considerable; yet when he didn't come first or make the A-grade team, Angus could only focus on what was missing in his son's performance. No doubt Michael felt deflated, angry and a failure. Just as Angus had with his own father.

The advent of serious illness often becomes the catalyst for us to resolve our inner difficulties. There is a sense of urgency and an increased willingness and determination to move forward. I am constantly amazed and inspired by people who, finding the courage within themselves, begin to heal dreadful traumas from the past or change lifelong patterns that have led only to misery. Angus began to see how the seeking of perfection in himself and in everyone else caused him – and them – so much pain.

Several months after our first meeting Angus decided to visit his father. He had realised that he and his father were very similar and, through knowing himself and what made him the person he was, had developed an understanding and compassion for his father. He felt there were things he needed to say to him. Angus knew that his father probably wouldn't recognise him nor perhaps be able to respond to him because his father was very frail and had long periods of dementia. We talked about what he felt he needed to say and I hoped that Angus's visit would bring some peace and resolution to their sense of separation and antagonism.

Gillian and Angus had resolved many of their difficulties and had grown closer. They functioned as a team working together rather than constantly pulling each other apart as they had during the first few weeks after his diagnosis. Gillian was enormously relieved and grateful for the change in Angus as the strained relationship between Michael and his father had caused her anguish. She had often felt sad and awkward as she tried to bolster Michael's self-esteem against the often unspoken, but nevertheless strongly felt criticism he received from his father. The atmosphere at home had lightened and Michael had joined Gillian in caring for his father, something Angus had railed against when he was first diagnosed.

The journey Angus made to his father's bedside was an exhausting one and he was relieved, on his arrival, to find his father asleep. His father had changed dramatically with the years and the effects Alzheimer's had produced.

Angus felt grateful that he didn't have to look into his father's eyes because he wasn't sure he'd be able to say the things in his heart if he felt any antagonism from him. He studied his father's hands instead, noting how different they were from his. His father had always been a practical man used to hard physical work, and his hands bore the scars of their use.

Angus sat by his bed for quite a while before he could bring himself to speak. He reflected for a long time on the way his father had always pushed him to better himself and not be someone who had to live by the use of his hands alone. Slowly he began to recount some of his childhood memories of the times they had spent together. Angus told him of the pain and hurt he felt when he couldn't get it right for his father, but he was also able to acknowledge the companionship that he had enjoyed with him. Angus shed tears as he thanked his father for the love he had shown him by pushing him to make a life of which he could be proud. Angus finally bent over his father to kiss him goodbye and, as he did, a tear slid from the corner of his father's eye. That single tear brought Angus completely undone and he sobbed with the tears of one long estranged from unconditional love.

A single healing moment can change the whole history of a relationship in a way that is both profound and miraculous. When we understand the truth of who we are and acknowledge, with respect, the journey we have made, we find a peace beyond the events of our lives and with the people who have been companions along our way.

VICKI

Many people struggle with the uncertainty of the future when they are faced with their own mortality. Frequently the future represents an anxiety which they feel cannot be discussed and this creates its own form of stress. Any serious illness can make a person irritable and unreasonable and this is usually directed towards the family more than anyone else. For a young person about to embark upon life as an adult, the advent of a life-threatening illness poses challenges that can be almost insurmountable.

Vicki had not long turned eighteen and had had a long drawn-out struggle with leukaemia. For her eighteenth birthday her parents had bought her a brand-new red car. She was enormously pleased and proud of this gift. To her it symbolised her ability to establish some independence away from home, something of which every young person dreams. For Vicki this was of paramount importance as for so many years, because of her illness, she had been more dependent upon her parents than most teenagers. As her illness progressed and she became very frail, it became quite impossible for her to drive the car. Her younger brother, Jeffrey, had just received his L plates and had decided he would maintain and care for her car as she was no longer able to do so.

Vicki became very sullen and irritable around about this time and particularly so towards Jeff, who reacted angrily to cover his hurt. This marred the whole atmosphere in the house and the rest of the family became irritable from the strain too.

Vicki's mother, Jan, asked me to visit the family and give Vicki a massage. We talked about the change in Vicki's spirits and the upset, hurt and confusion felt by her family as she seemed to be rejecting them. We hoped that some quiet time spent with me might enable Vicki to speak what was in her heart.

Massage can be a wonderful therapy. It creates a warm and safe environment in which neither the person giving the massage nor the person receiving the massage need talk unless they want to. On my first visit I was very much aware that Vicki was feeling me out, even though I was the one giving her the massage! When I finished massaging her, she asked if I would return in a couple of days' time.

During the massage on my second visit, Vicki gave me a key to unlock her distress. Her brother was outside washing her car and started it up to move it closer to the garden tap. Vicki's body tensed and it was obvious something had upset her, yet she still tried to conceal it. On gentle investigation the problem she was having became obvious. She became very angry and said, 'Petrea, he can't even wait until I'm dead', then she curled up in my arms and sobbed. Vicki's thinking may seem convoluted, but someone who is sick has an unlimited amount of time to cogitate over things and perhaps blow them out of proportion or distort them.

Vicki believed Jeff was taking such good care of her car because he knew that, very likely, he was going to get it should she die. To her family, and especially to Jeff, this couldn't have been further from the truth. His motivations were clear – it was his way of showing she could rely on him to take care of her prized possession until she was able to resume those responsibilities herself. In her mind there was no such honourable intention.

When the family could see this from her rather distorted viewpoint, they were able to reassure Vicki and make some simple adjustments to solve the problem. Jeff found a beautiful key-case and had it engraved with her initials; and instead of him keeping the keys, which he had retained up until now, he would go to her and ask if she'd like him to polish the car for her or turn over the engine, always returning the keys to her afterwards. In this way, the explosiveness went out of the situation and the household settled down again to the warm and open place it was before.

We often avoid talking about things which we find difficult for fear that we will upset ourselves and those we love. By withholding our fears, however, we deny ourselves the possibility of communicating deeply with those who truly love and want to support us. Vicki's family took the opportunity to open up the painful conversations that needed to take place so that she could explore with them her fears, concepts and uncertainties about death and dying.

Several weeks passed and then Vicki asked her mother to have an identical key-case engraved with Jeff's initials. A few days before she died, Vicki called Jeff to her bedside and gave him the keys to her car. She chided him about not 'becoming a hoon' and told him she would watch over him always.

RAY

I believe that at some level, even when we are seemingly deeply unconscious, there is a part of us that has a great awareness. This belief has been confirmed many times and Ray's story illustrates it well.

The first time Ray came to the support group at the Albion Street Centre in Sydney he told us he had immigrated to Australia many years before, but now, because of his illness, he longed for his family roots. He felt trapped by his feelings because he knew that his family wouldn't be able to cope with his illness because he had AIDS.

Ray's family lived in a little village in Wales and he knew only too well how homophobic the townspeople could be. He hadn't told his parents that he was ill because he was afraid that his elderly mother would want to visit him and perhaps even stay on to care for him. On the one hand Ray ached for the kind of caring he felt she could extend – including her delicious dumplings – yet on the other hand he knew she would have great difficulty accepting his friends and lifestyle. Besides, he was afraid that his illness and the travelling would be the death of her.

The thought of never seeing his parents again made Ray feel very isolated and alone. He said he fluctuated between wanting to outlive his parents so that they need never know of the 'shame of his disease and lifestyle', and wanting to die now because he found his loneliness and the fact that he felt his life was a sham intolerable. He knew his parents loved him, but they didn't know he was gay, and he felt that might get in the way of them loving him. This had been the main reason for him immigrating to Australia.

Depression hung about Ray like a soggy blanket. His eyes were lifeless; his shoulders stooped, and he dragged himself around as if he was on his last legs – which he wasn't. His health was quite good, in fact, and were it not for his engulfing depression he perhaps had many years of life left in him.

Two weeks after I met Ray I received a note in the mail with a key. My heart sank as I read his words. *By the time you receive this note I will be dead. I'm sorry to do this to you but I can't think of any other way.* Ray had included some contact details for his family and friends. I called one of his friends and arranged to meet her at his apartment. As I unlocked his door every part of me wanted to be somewhere else.

Ray was not dead, but he was close to it. We called an ambulance who delivered him to hospital, and after two or three days he was alert enough for me to visit. He looked more miserable than ever and lamented the fact that his suicide attempt had been worse than futile. He now had serious complications from having lain in a very awkward position for two days. These complications to his circulation, plus his intentions to end his life, kept him in hospital for several weeks.

During that time I visited him at least twice a week. Gradually his outlook improved and he chose to spend more time with the other men in the AIDS ward. Some of them were practically boys, only in their early twenties, and Ray found it a tragedy that they should die before they had really had any life. He gradually took it upon himself to buy for them books, magazines and other luxuries they couldn't afford.

One of the conditions of Ray's release from hospital was that he regularly attend our support group. Gradually his view of life shifted to a more positive one as he became more immersed in the gay community, especially with those who shared his illness. He volunteered for one of the programs which offered practical support for people living with AIDS and, though he would now always walk with a stick, Ray would visit someone in their home if they were lonely or too ill to go out. He also attended several of our residential programs in the country, frequently driving others who were too sick or didn't have cars, and became involved in our CLOWN project. Throughout all this Ray continued to deliver magazines to the young patients in the AIDS ward and to run errands for them.

When we begin to focus on the needs of others we

often find that our own load becomes lighter. This was certainly true for Ray.

Over the next few years Ray wrote many loving letters to his parents and, though he kept from them the details of his illness, he told them that he was gay. He wept as he read their response to the support group. They wrote that they had always known he was 'different' from other boys and, though they didn't feel any need to understand his lifestyle, they had always loved him and would continue to do so. Not long after he received this letter Ray's parents died within a few weeks of each other.

Ray shared with the group his sadness and grief at their deaths but far greater was his deep satisfaction that all that needed to be said between them had been done. He felt liberated by the thought that his parents knew who he was and loved him, and that his death would not now cause them any distress.

About this time Ray asked me to be with him when he died. I said I'd certainly be there if it was at all possible.

Some weeks later Ray was hospitalised for the last time and I visited him as often as I could. The staff telephoned me at three one Sunday morning and suggested I come immediately to the hospital if I wanted to be with him when he died.

I arrived half an hour later and Ray greeted me warmly. With great effort he reached up so that we could hug one another, and I pulled up a chair.

For several hours Ray seemed very peaceful and content as he gradually moved beyond words. His breathing was regular and his eyes were often focused on mine. I felt a deep sense of connection with him and there was a companionable silence around us that I suspect we both found comforting.

At about one that afternoon a nurse called me to the desk and told me that a friend of Ray's had just rung to say that he was on his way to the hospital to say goodbye. Ray had spoken occasionally of this man and it was clear to me that he didn't think of him as a friend at all.

When I told Ray that this person was on his way to the hospital and would be there in about twenty minutes, I suspected that one of two things would happen. Ray would either die very quickly or he would become deeply unconscious so that he would not 'be there' when this man arrived.

Within five minutes Ray's eyes fluttered closed and his breathing became very regular as he went into deep unconsciousness. I have seen this many times and it seems to me that the person's body goes onto automatic pilot whilst their 'spirit' is elsewhere. Their breathing becomes very regular, almost mechanical, and I always have the strong impression that though their body is there and warm to the touch, their spirit is actually off somewhere else.

The 'friend' came, said his goodbyes and left without any change in Ray's condition. For a further hour Ray remained deeply unconscious. By this time, I was aware of the fact that I was due to lecture that afternoon at four o'clock at a conference for HIV-positive women. I would need to leave the hospital at least half an hour before I was due to lecture. It was now three o'clock. It's awful to feel that you want a person to hurry up and die, yet I was beginning to feel torn between my two commitments.

I took Ray's hand in mine and told him my dilemma. 'Ray, I have a lecture to give in one hour and I need to leave here in half an hour in order to make it.'

Ray's breathing immediately changed as his eyes opened and once again focused on mine. 'You're back!' I said. 'It's nice to see you. It's OK for you to go now. I'm with you.'

I took on Ray's breathing pattern as a way of connecting more deeply with him. During the next half hour Ray stopped breathing three times. Each time his eyes would remain focused on mine and I would talk to him quietly about letting go, that everything was alright, that he was safe and loved. At one stage I suggested to him that he might see a light or his parents who had died a few weeks previously. His gaze shifted from my eyes to somewhere just to my right and his whole being seemed to soften and let go. The look on his face was beautiful, as if he had seen something which moved him to the core of his being. His gaze finally shifted back to my eyes as he let go his last breath with ease.

The contrast between Ray's first attempt at death and his final letting go was certainly not lost on me. I felt grateful for the peace he had found and the courage he had shown in meeting the obstacles to that peace along the way.

Ray left his body two minutes before I left for my lecture. Two strong impressions remained with me. One, he certainly seemed to have consciously *left* his body; and two, having completed a good life, well lived, he chose the timing and the manner of his departure.

ANNE-MARIE

When we grow weary of trying to deal with a difficult situation we can begin to question or lose faith in our beliefs. These beliefs may have helped us through many difficulties and challenges in the past and may have formed the foundation upon which we have lived our life. It can be devastating to find that they no longer serve us.

Anne-Marie attended our support and meditation groups for over six years. She was enormously loving and compassionate to all who came to our groups and she had formed deep friendships born of shared experiences with many of the participants. Her cancer was slowly but relentlessly taking over her pancreas and liver, and this led to many digestive complications.

She had been a religious sister since she was in her teens and her faith in the Gospel was central to every aspect of her life. As her health declined she experienced depression for the first time in her life. Her doctors told her that this depression was chemical in nature, caused by the advancement of her disease. However, this was hard for her to comprehend because the feelings were so powerful and felt so real that where they came from was irrelevant.

When Anne-Marie could no longer attend the group I used to visit her at the convent. On one occasion I found her distraught and tearful. She told me she had completely lost her faith in God and that this made a mockery of her life's work. She had believed that if she loved God and gave her life to Him, He would never give her something beyond her ability to cope with – and He had. She no longer wanted to struggle with her body and she felt defeated by forces that she could neither resist nor comprehend. She felt angry and badly done by and seemed to relish the words, 'It's not fair!' rolling off her lips when previously they had only spoken words of love and forgiveness.

I was saddened by her words because, to me, she lived the very essence of her beliefs. However, the feelings she was describing were ones that I was familiar with and I told Anne-Marie a story about a crucifix in the town of Sorrento in Italy.

For a couple of months before I went to Assisi and the monastery there, I lived in Sorrento. Right in the heart of the town there was a beautiful cathedral. In truth, it wasn't actually beautiful in the architectural sense of the word. But I loved the huge cavern of quietness within the building. The contrast between the bustle of life outside and the serenity inside always struck me. I spent most of my days within the cathedral meditating and praying. The locals got quite used to my presence there and I was usually oblivious to the masses being conducted around me.

At the back of one of the side chapels inside the cathedral there stood an enormous crucifix, perhaps two metres high. It was black with age and lack of care. One day I asked the priest if I could clean it. He knew I had leukaemia and he was concerned that I might be taking on too much, but I convinced him that it would be excellent therapy and so my labour of love began.

With a toothbrush, a tin of Brasso and a soft cloth, I began at the very top of the cross. A glint of gold appeared and I realised with delight that the cross was made of brass. Each day I worked quietly in the back of the cathedral, out of sight of most people, except for those who were fond of that particular chapel. The cathedral was locked up each day between twelve and four for the afternoon siesta. Most days I would secrete myself away somewhere in the cathedral so that I'd be locked in for those hours undisturbed.

As I cleaned the thorns pressed into the head of Jesus I wept knowing the terrible pain we human beings inflict upon one another out of fear and judgement. When I gently removed all the dirt from around the nails penetrating his hands I was moved by his willingness to sacrifice everything for his truth. Surely he must have doubted his faith as he clambered up the hill carrying the cross. If he had no doubt, then I am beyond hope. If we share in our doubt and choose to trust anyway, then we are all saved. Surely Anne-Marie's doubts and despair were no different from those He too had felt.

Each day as I cleaned I journeyed within myself, and my meditations upon the story detailed in the Gospels deepened and expanded. It took two months of daily cleaning to bring the crucifix to its full glory. It shone like a beacon of hope and the priests gave it a new place of prominence near the altar of the cathedral where it still stands.

It sometimes takes a lifetime to bring us to our full glory. The events of our lives can be the catalyst by which we shed all that stands in the way of our light. Then we can serve as a beacon to remind each other of the love and light that dwells within.

Anne-Marie listened quietly as I told her my story. Her eyes had filled with tears which flowed down her cheeks unchecked as she was touched by those parts of my story which connected with her. I left her alone with her thoughts and promised to visit her the following day.

The challenge of losing one's independence and dignity is hard for anyone and this had contributed to Anne-Marie's resentment of her body and its illness.

Anne-Marie was hospitalised the following day and I had the opportunity of sitting with her in her final hours. When I arrived at her bedside she grasped my hand and the look of serenity on her face made unnecessary any conversation about her previous struggles of faith.

A PATH TO PEACE

These stories are my answer to those who would ask the question, 'Why do you work with the dying?' We are all embarked upon the journey of our own healing, to reconnect with the parts of ourselves that we've long hidden from our own, and perhaps other peoples, view.

I believe that in all of us there resides beauty, truth, love and goodness. For some it becomes a lifelong passion to know the real depths of those qualities within us. Each experience becomes an opportunity to test ourselves against what *is* in order to understand who we are and to bring to full manifestation that which aches in us for fulfilment. We can learn not to take the events of our lives so personally. They are simply opportunities to grow in wisdom and in love.

It can take a lifetime to find this fulfilment. We each

only have moment by moment to live our lives. When we live with awareness in each moment then we can look back on a lifetime full of being present to life's richness and depth.

The people within these pages have been pushed to their edge. They've been confronted with the unimaginable and the uninvited. Through these events they have found their healing.

We are living in a time when we're all being pushed to our edge. We've lost faith in the institutions that once formed the structure upon which we conducted our lives. We struggle to look with admiration and respect to our governments, judiciary, politicians, medical and educational systems, churches or economy. The foundations of our society as we know it are crumbling. We have raped and pillaged Mother Earth and she too is struggling to find her balance.

The people within these covers have found their disease presents them with an opportunity for self-exploration and understanding. We can learn much from them. We don't need to have a life-threatening disease in order to commit ourselves to this deep and profound healing.

We are essential to one another because no finer mirror exists to clarify who we are than those people we're blessed to know. They reflect back to us our ability, or lack of it, to be wholly present, open and loving and compassionate to one another. Each of us must take responsibility for our own healing. Then we will more easily find a path to peace and healing within our families, our communities, our countries and our world.

THE PETREA KING QUEST FOR LIFE CENTRE

At the Petrea King Quest for Life Centre, we give people practical strategies for living well in challenging circumstances and for finding meaning in the midst of life's unexpected events. We recognise that we can't always change what happens to us in life but we can play an active role in how we're going to respond to what happens to us. We value peace of mind above all else.

There are many events in life that stop us in our tracks and cause us to consider how best to meet the challenge we face: an unexpected diagnosis, accident, loss or tragedy can be such an impetus.

Some people seek more meaningful ways of managing the challenging circumstances of chronic illness, multiple loss, anxiety, relationship breakdown, depression or the con-sequences of past abuse. Other people choose to take time-out to review their life with the intention of deepening their relationship with themselves and living a more satisfying and meaningful life in the future.

Since 1985 more than 50,000 people have attended residential programs or counselling with Petrea and her team of trained health professionals.

Since 1999 our residential programs and services have been conducted at the Quest for Life Centre – an historic guesthouse set in 3.6 tranquil hectares of gardens at Bundanoon, in the beautiful Southern Highlands of New South Wales.

Our programs endeavour to support each participant to regain a sense of control over their lives and actively participate in their own healing. Each person leaves with a greater understanding of themselves and a deeper respect for their unique story. Content of the programs is tailored to the people attending each program and varies accordingly. Programs include the following five areas:

Techniques for living in the present

- Relaxation, visualisation and meditation techniques
- Living the life you came here to live
- Transforming adversity; learning to respond, not react

Mind–body connection

- The science of stress and illness
- Creating an environment for healing
- Harnessing the power of the mind
- The role of intuition

Managing thoughts and emotions

- Peace of mind: what it is and how to attain and maintain it
- Understanding the power of the mind to create and counter stress
- Forgiveness and getting 'up to date'
- What is a positive attitude; how to attain and maintain it

Complementary advice supporting medical treatment

- Natural therapies to help with pain, sleep, symptoms and side effects
- Practical advice on diet

Moving on from here

- Rearranging priorities
- Enhancing communication, resilience, relationship
- Getting back in the driver's seat of life
- Learning to live skillfully with stress and move beyond difficult emotions

If you feel we can assist you through one of our residential programs or other services, please call us with your particular needs. We look forward to our paths crossing with yours.

The Quest for Life Foundation

The Petrea King Quest for Life Centre is owned and operated by the Quest for Life Foundation, a registered charity established in 1990 by Petrea King.

The Quest for Life Foundation subsidises all programs as well as an additional subsidy with the support of the NSW Health Department for people on pensions and low incomes.

Donations assist us to support the provision and expansion of our services and are fully tax deductible.

Petrea King Quest for Life Centre
Ph: (61 2) 4883 6599
PO Box 390
Bundanoon NSW 2578
Australia
Email: info@questforlife.org.au
Web:www.questforlife.org.au

Petrea King Products

Much of life is spent taking on more information, more identities and more learning. We then identify who we are by what we do. In meditation we unveil the treasure of our human 'being' beyond our human 'doing'.

As we quieten the chatter of our minds we discover an inner wellspring from which intuition, joy, inspiration, imagination, wisdom and contentment more effortlessly flow. Meditation becomes that sacred space in which we replenish and refresh ourselves.

Your life matters. You are not here by chance. You are here to make the journey of your life by taking responsibility for your physical, mental, emotional and spiritual wellbeing. My books and meditation practices detail practical ways in which you can reclaim your life and establish peace of mind. I trust they will assist you in creating health, happiness and harmony in your life.

Relaxation and Meditation Practices

Available as MP3 audio files at:
https://shop.questforlife.org.au/meditations/

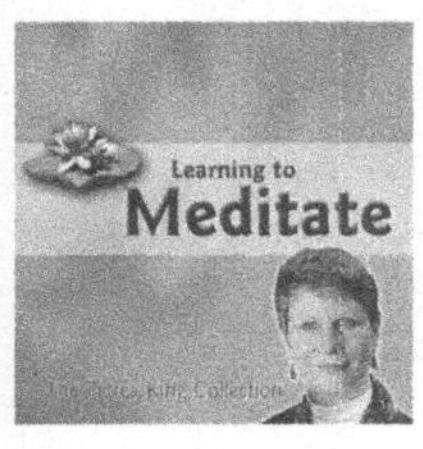

Learning to Meditate (New Version 2004)

This title combines an excellent explanation of meditation with a guided progressive relaxation and meditation practice with Petrea.

You will learn what meditation is and how to practise it. You will understand when and why to practise meditation, how the mind works and how to manage it more effectively.

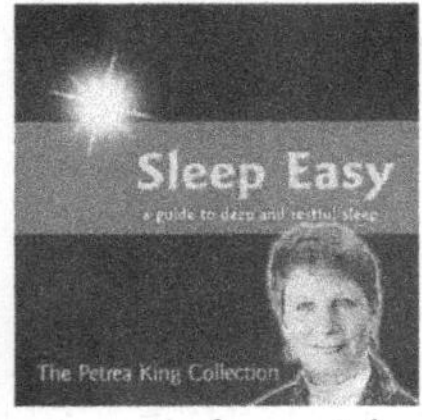

Sleep (formerly Sleep Easy)

No-one has ever heard the end of this practice! Designed to guide you into deep and restful sleep, it is ideal for the chronic insomniac or people having temporary difficulty with sleeping. You are guided through a progressive relaxation then into a beautiful garden of peace where sleep will overtake you. The CD comes with a bonus booklet of tips from Petrea for developing good sleep habits.

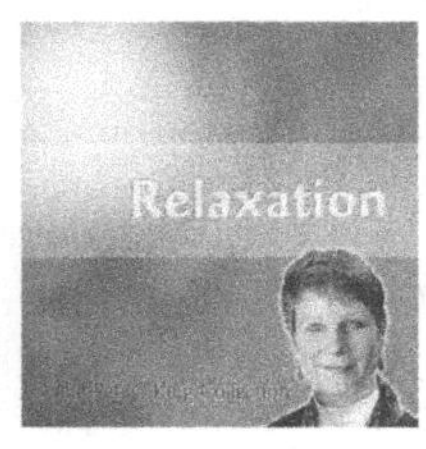

Relaxation

A guided relaxation to release stress and increase immune function. We imagine we're at the beach, where we put all our stresses in a rainbow hot air balloon and release it. We enter the water and, floating on our back, bathe in the golden light of the sun and feel its healing energy. After a brief meditation we return refreshed and energised. Plus the relaxing silver flute music of Gopal.

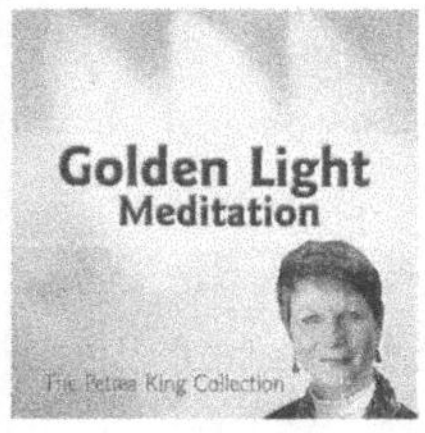

Golden Light Meditation

Petrea guides you through a progressive relaxation and uses golden light imagery through the body to create a powerful environment for physical, emotional and spiritual healing. After a brief meditation we return refreshed and energised. Plus the beautiful healing music of *Windsong* by Phil Colville.

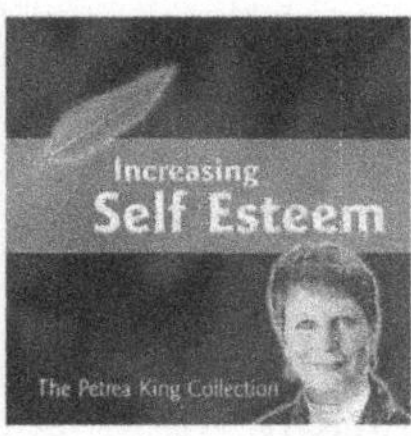

Increasing Self Esteem

Petrea talks about what makes or damages self-esteem and how we can improve our self-confidence. We are guided deep into the rainforest where there's a waterfall cascading into a peaceful pool of water and visualise ourselves living with all the qualities we want in our life. This practice is helpful in changing negative attitudes or for goal-setting and is a favourite with teenagers and adults.

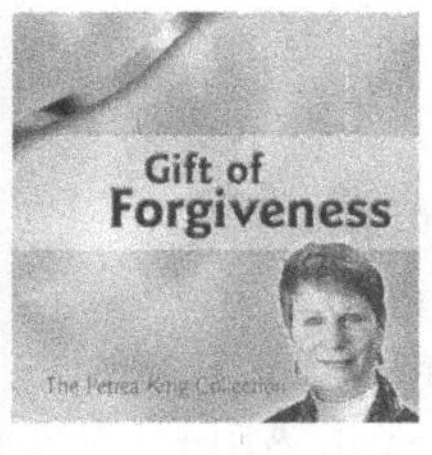

Gift of Forgiveness

Through extending compassionate self-forgiveness we can enter a deeper relationship with ourselves and others built on self-understanding. In these two practices Petrea guides you through a progressive relaxation, then using imagery to connect with the qualities of our inner child we extend forgiveness to ourselves and others.

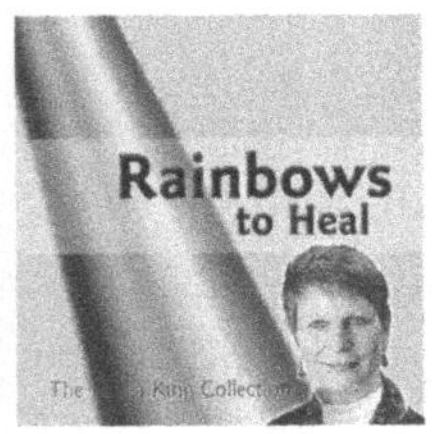

Rainbows to Heal

Petrea guides you through a progressive relaxation and self-healing practice that uses imagery to fill your energy centres with the colours of the rainbow. A second practice involves extending the colours of the rainbow to bring love or healing to another person or situation.

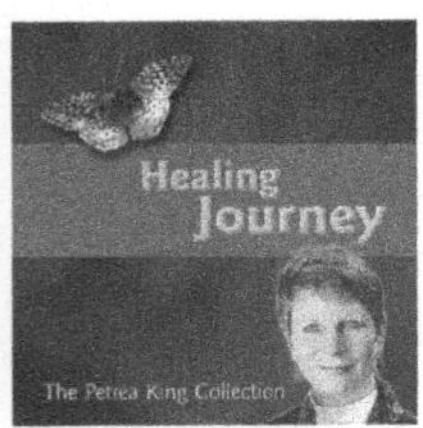

Healing Journey

Petrea guides you through a progressive relaxation and into a beautiful garden where water and light bring about peace and healing. After a brief meditation we return refreshed and energised. This is an ideal practice for those who want to create wellness, inner peace, strength and self-confidence. Plus the beautiful healing music of *Windsong* by Phil Colville.

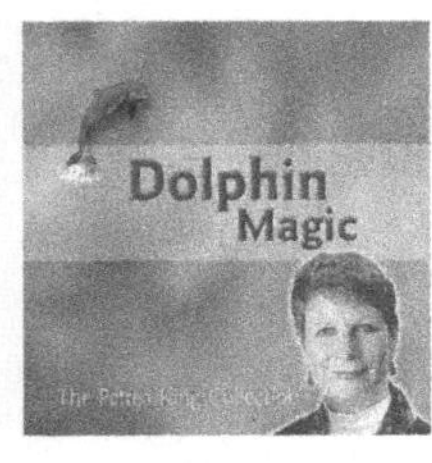

Dolphin Magic

Journey deep beneath the sea with your own special dolphin to a crystal cavern full of the colours of the rainbow. Allow the colours to wash through your body to bring feelings of peace and renewal. After a healing meditation you return to the surface with your dolphin, refreshed and energised. Plus the beautiful healing music of *Earthsea* by Phil Colville.

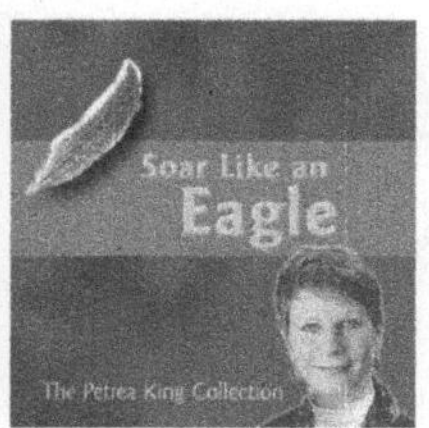

Soar Like an Eagle

High on a mountaintop at sunset you relax and enjoy the peace and serenity before floating effortlessly as an eagle. Entering a meditation you absorb the qualities of self-confidence, strength, wisdom and clarity and return refreshed and energised. Plus the beautiful healing music of *Solis* by Phil Colville.

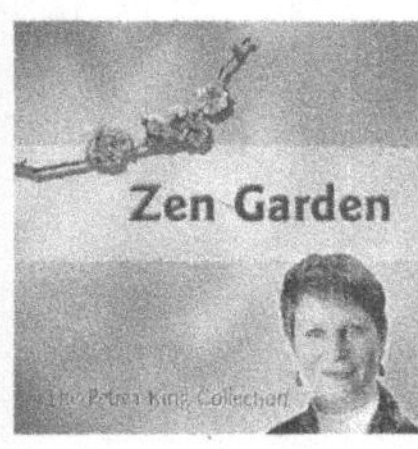

Zen Garden

A beautiful relaxation and meditation practice set in a garden full of cherry blossoms. We meet our wise inner being by a pool of water and ask for the gift of a quality we need or the answer to a question. We return refreshed and energised, bringing back with us what we need. Plus the beautiful silver flute music of Gopal.

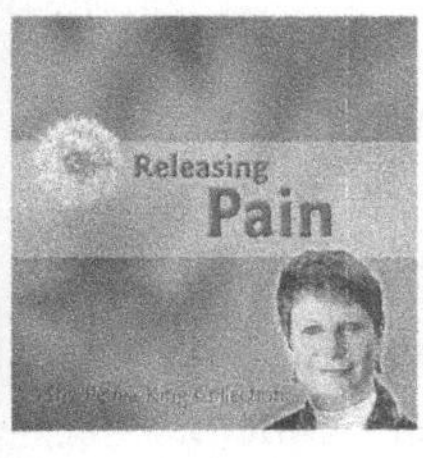

Releasing Pain

Using progressive relaxation and imagery to release physical, mental and emotional pain, Petrea guides you through a relaxation and the practice of Yoga Nidra to effectively manage and release pain.

Books by Petrea

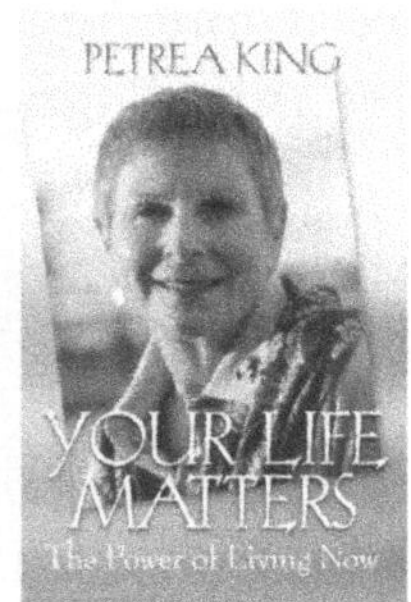

Your Life Matters: The Power of Living Now

Your Life Matters is a guide to establishing peace of mind, and living an authentic and fulfilling life. In this wise, necessary and practical book, Petrea King teaches us how to live from the inside out rather than the outside in. By sharing her many principles and guidelines to developing our sense of self, treating our bodies right and adapting to life's challenges, Petrea shows us the way to peace and all-round health and wellbeing.

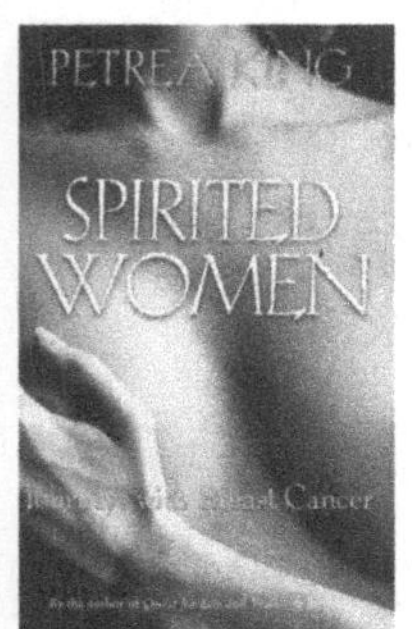

Spirited Women: Journeys with Breast Cancer

Spirited Women addresses the many practical issues women face when diagnosed with breast cancer. The book has quotes from hundreds of women who describe their diverse reactions to things such as diagnosis, choosing doctors, confronting their scars, sexuality and body image, talking to children, living with uncertainty, dealing with recurrence, facing death, letting go, resolving the past and learning to live more abundantly and peacefully in the present. In addition, there is a wealth of practical information that educates and empowers those whose lives are touched by breast cancer.

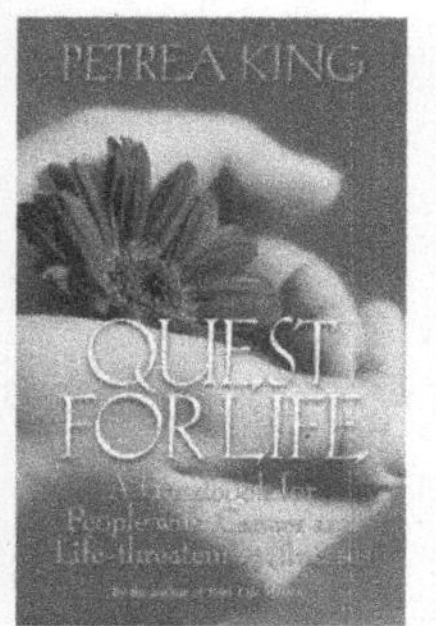

Quest for Life: Living Well with Cancer and Life-threatening Illnesses

This bestseller is an essential handbook for anyone with cancer and for those who love or care for them. It is the story of Petrea's recovefrom leukaemia combined with the practical knowledge gained from working with tens of thousands of individuals with cancer and other life-challenging illnesses.

In *Quest for Life* Petrea provides accessible guidelines for combining the best of medical care with commonsense lifestyle practices and naturopathic advice – all based on Petrea's training in health, healing and meditation.

Further information or to order these products:

Petrea King
PO Box 190
Bundanoon NSW 2578
Australia
Ph: (61 2) 4883 6805
Fax: (61 2) 4883 6632
Email: info@petreaking.com
Web: www.petreaking.com